Issues in ophthalmic practice

Issues in ophthalmic practice:
Current and future challenges

Edited by Susan Watkinson

Issues in Ophthalmic Practice: Current and future challenges
Susan Watkinson

ISBN: 978-1-905539-17-8

First published 2009

British Library Cataloguing in Publication Data
A catalogue record for this book is available from the British Library

Notice
Clinical practice and medical knowledge constantly evolve. Standard safety precautions must be followed, but, as knowledge is broadened by research, changes in practice, treatment and drug therapy may become necessary or appropriate. Readers must check the most current product information provided by the manufacturer of each drug to be administered and verify the dosages and correct administration, as well as contraindications. It is the responsibility of the practitioner, utilising the experience and knowledge of the patient, to determine dosages and the best treatment for each individual patient. Any brands mentioned in this book are as examples only and are not endorsed by the Publisher. Neither the Publisher nor the authors assume any liability for any injury and/or damage to persons or property arising from this publication.

The Publisher
To contact M&K Publishing write to:
M&K Update Ltd · The Old Bakery · St. John's Street
Keswick · Cumbria CA12 5AS
Tel: 01768 773030 · Fax: 01768 781099
publishing@mkupdate.co.uk
www.mkupdate.co.uk

Designed and typeset by Mary Blood
Printed in UK by Ferguson Print, Keswick.

Contents

Figures and tables

Contributors

Susan Watkinson, BA, RN, OND (Hons), PGCEA, MSc (University of Surrey), PhD (University of Surrey), is a Senior Lecturer in Adult Nursing, Faculty of Health and Human Sciences, Thames Valley University, Slough, UK. She qualified as an ophthalmic nurse at Moorfields Eye Hospital where she also held Sister and Clinical Teaching posts. Ophthalmic nursing remains her specialist clinical interest and she has published extensively within this field. She gained an MSc in Educational Studies and a PhD in Education from the University of Surrey. She has considerable experience of teaching ophthalmic nursing, research, ethics and philosophy within pre- and post-registration nurse education.

Anthony Afanu, RN, BSc (Hons) Professional Practice with Ophthalmic Nursing, is a Senior Staff Nurse in the Oxford Eye Hospital, Lichfield Specialist Day Surgery Unit. His specialist interest is in ophthalmic day surgery, and coaching and mentoring.

Paul Buka, MIHM, MSc (University of Leicester), PGCE, LL.B (Hons), FETC (City & Guilds 7307), HNC (Public Admin), RN, is a Senior Lecturer in Adult Nursing, Faculty of Health and Human Sciences, Thames Valley University, London, UK. He read law for his first degree, specialising in Healthcare Law and Crime and subsequently gained a master's degree in Criminal Justice and Criminology. As well as experience in teaching adult nursing, with a special interest in Healthcare Law and Ethics, he has taught Law in FE and has publications in the area of Healthcare Law and Ethics.

Kathleen Chambers, RN, RM, RMN, Cert Ed, BSc, MA, is a retired Senior Lecturer of the Faculty of Health and Human Sciences, Thames Valley University, London, UK. Her specialist clinical interests are neonatal nursing and child law. She gained an MA in Child Care Law and Practice from the University of Keele. She has considerable experience of teaching Child Law and Child Protection within pre- and post-registration nurse education.

Lavona Dampies, RGN, RM, Diploma in Operating Theatre Nursing Sciences, BSc (Hons) Professional Practice with Ophthalmic Nursing, is a Clinical Lead Practitioner in the ophthalmic theatre at the Royal Berkshire Hospital NHS Foundation Trust, Reading, UK. She has extensive experience as an ophthalmic theatre nurse and is currently studying for an MA in Leading, Managing and Partnership Working. She has also recently been teaching students undertaking the CPPD in Ophthalmic Nursing course at Thames Valley University.

Ramesh Seewoodhary, BSc (Hons) Biological Sciences, RGN, OND (Hons) FETC 730, Intensive Care Certificate JBCNS, RCNT, RNT, Cert. Ed., is a Senior Lecturer in Adult Nursing, Thames Valley University, Slough, UK. His clinical interests and expertise are within ophthalmic nursing, particularly in the field of Accident and Emergency eye care and primary care, applied physiology, and mentorship. He has published extensively within the field of ophthalmic nursing and has acted as nursing adviser to nursing journals.

Foreword

Ophthalmic nursing is becoming increasingly complex and specialised as an area of care and yet it comprises the very essence of caring practice. The past three decades have heralded major advances in the management and care of people with ophthalmic conditions, in all age groups. The publication of this book is timely as it represents the most current, evidence-based practice in ophthalmic nursing care. But this book is more than a wealth of information related to the nursing management of people with various ophthalmic conditions; it also succeeds in being an interactive, consciousness-raising text that will enable ophthalmic practitioners through reflective practice to consider critically the wider issues in their everyday practice. Ophthalmic nurses need to continue to develop the habits of critical thought as a way of maintaining themselves within a wider community of practice. This book will play a major role in that endeavour.

What makes this book particularly unique is its blend of clinical care with wider political and professional issues underpinning day-to-day ophthalmic care. The editor and individual authors have created chapters related to all aspects of ophthalmic practice in a way that enables the reader to raise their understanding of the changing nature of ophthalmic nursing, including changing demographics, the role of evidence and research in ophthalmic nursing, technological advances in ophthalmic care and the need for ophthalmic nurses to engage in continuing professional development. The integration of evidence-based ophthalmic practice is leading to tremendous improvements and advancements in the care of patients, in all settings, with ophthalmic disorders.

Professor Diane Marks-Maran
Visiting Professor of Nursing, Kingston University

Preface

This text will highlight the ongoing effects of national healthcare policy on ophthalmic care delivery, while exploring the implications and impact of such changes. Ophthalmic nurse practitioners face current issues as well as future challenges for the 21st century on a day-to-day basis. These are considered to be the outcome of not only demographic change, advancing technology and research, but also of increasing government legislation.

The target group for this text is mainly ophthalmic nurse practitioners and allied healthcare professionals. Other healthcare professionals will however be able to have a better insight into this specialist area. It is not intended to be a 'how to do' text. On the contrary, it has been written to encourage its readers to engage in the process of thinking critically about the most significant influences impacting on current practice from professional, national, socio-economic, as well as legal and ethical issues. Such issues will undoubtedly present ophthalmic practitioners with many challenges for the future.

The author and contributors to this book challenge readers to respond by becoming more pro-active in devising strategies for addressing these current issues and for meeting with inevitable future challenges.

Acknowledgements

The author would like to thank all those involved in the production process, especially my commissioning editor, Mike Roberts. I also acknowledge the valuable contributions from Anthony Afanu, Ramesh Seewoodhary, Lavona Dampies, Paul Buka, and Kathy Chambers in respect of Chapters 2, 3, 4, 5, 6, 7, 8, and 9.

I also wish to thank both my academic and clinical colleagues for their continued moral support during the writing of this book. Special thanks to Eileen Scott, my critical friend, for her painstaking review of several of my chapters.

Chapter 1
Introduction:
Issues in ophthalmic practice – current and future challenges
Susan Watkinson

Demographic changes
Technological changes
Ocular disease in the UK
Care and service provision
The future role of the ophthalmic practitioner

Introduction

The main aims of this book are to discuss some of the important issues faced by ophthalmic practitioners in the United Kingdom (UK) on a day-to-day basis, and to explore the current and future challenges posed by such issues for the delivery of ophthalmic care for the 21st century. National issues are considered to be the outcome of demographic change, advancing technology and research, increased government health legislation, the rising incidence of ocular disease, the increasing complexity surrounding legal and ethical practice, and the need for life-long learning and professional competence. Local issues have recently been highlighted as bureaucracy, staff shortages, poor management and lack of leadership, absence of appropriate training and induction, and difficulties with recruitment and retention leading to overuse of temporary staff (DoH, 2008). Poor communication skills, insufficient motivation, and lack of reflection on practice may also be justifiably added to this list. In any event, these issues translate into significant constraints for practitioners at local level, especially when trying to meet the government's targets for effective and high quality delivery of care (DoH, 2008). However, whether national or local, such issues will inevitably impact on the delivery of ophthalmic care for the 21st century, and the expectations of the future role of the ophthalmic practitioner in achieving this.

The exploration of such issues and challenges within ophthalmic healthcare delivery constitutes the main thrust of this text and also determines the scope and remit of discussion within the forthcoming chapters. This text is aimed primarily at ophthalmic practitioners and allied healthcare professionals. However, visual problems are undoubtedly a universal phenomenon and will trigger debate and pose many healthcare challenges for the future. For this reason, other healthcare professionals will profit from reading and engaging with the discussion to gain a better insight into the particular issues within this specialist area. Raising the consciousness of the readers of this text is important as early detection and diagnosis of sight-threatening ocular disease, and effective treatment to eliminate or control the loss of sight constitute some of the major challenges for the future role of the ophthalmic practitioner in the UK.

This chapter will now present an overview of the demographic and technological changes taking place and discuss the impact of such changes on current and future ophthalmic practice. We will then discuss the main ocular diseases prevalent in the UK with reference to aetiological and epidemiological factors. The implications of ocular disease for the care of the visually impaired will consequently be explored. The impact of·recent government policies and National Service Frameworks on healthcare delivery will then be discussed. This chapter concludes by outlining the important future role of the ophthalmic practitioner with reference to the recent recommendations provided in the Darzi Report (DoH, 2008). At this stage, the reader is invited to participate in two key Thinking Points as a means of triggering the process of reflection and critical thinking about the current situation.

Demographic Changes

Demographic changes

Sight loss is largely an age-related phenomenon (DoH, 2001). Worldwide, there are currently approximately 180 million people with a visual disability. Of these, up to 45 million are blind (WHO, 1999). Overall, approximately 4% of people aged 60 years and above are thought to be blind, and 60% of them live in Sub-

Saharan Africa, China and India. For the future, the age distribution of the world population is set to undergo marked changes due to demographic transition and the long-term effects of fertility reduction (UNPD 2002). This means that by the middle of the 21st century the number of older people will outnumber the number of children at the global level (UNPD 2002). Statistics indicate that globally, the number of people aged over 60 will more than triple, increasing from 606 million today to nearly 2 billion by 2050. The increase in the number of the oldest, those aged over 80, is expected to be even more marked, increasing from 69 million in 2000 to 379 million in 2050 (UNPD 2002). In view of this predicted demographic transition, not only will the burden of ocular disease and sight loss increase, but also the need to provide appropriate eye care services will increase worldwide, particularly in the developing countries.

The situation in the United Kingdom also reflects these predicted global trends. Indeed, currently, 70% of all people with sight problems in this country are aged 65 and over (DoH, 2001). It is estimated that by 2025, one-fifth of the UK population, that is, 12.8 million people, will be over the age of 65, and, similar to predictions worldwide, it is expected that the number of people aged 80 and above will grow fastest to reach 3.5 million by the year 2025. Furthermore, it is in this age group that the serious sight problems will be experienced.

In relation to children, by 2050 there will be one child for every five people (UNPD 2002). In the United Kingdom, in 2001, there were 14.8 million children aged under 20. Although there has been little change in the proportion of younger people under the age of 20, there were relatively fewer under-5-year-olds and 15-to-19-year-olds in 2001 compared with 1990. The 2001 Census showed that for the first time there was a lower proportion of children aged below 16 than people aged 60 and over (Office for National Statistics (ONS), 2008). However, as international migration is projected to remain high during the twenty-first century, the UK can expect to see a continued growth in the proportion of children in ethnic minority groups (UNPD 2002). Between 1992 and 2000 the overall growth was mainly in the Black-African (37%), Black Mixed (49%), and Bangladeshi (30%) ethnic groups. The most important implication of this is the need for ocular health education to be provided to such groups.

However, one of the fundamental challenges here for practitioners is effective communication, since language barriers may exist within the immigrant population.

Technological changes

Technological changes

Clearly, the relationship between a predicted demographic transition and technological change is an important one. The need for health technology is governed by demographic, aetiological and epidemiological factors. Indeed, future mortality and morbidity depends on how well health technology can make a reduction in infant mortality, accidents at all ages, as well as major systemic diseases such as diabetes mellitus.

Technological advance signals current and future challenges for ophthalmic nurse practitioners. In the UK, for example, survival rates for pre-term babies have increased significantly over the last 40 years, from approximately 5% to 65% for babies with birth weight less than 1000g and from approximately 35% to 90% for those between 1000g and 1500g birth weight. As a result, the number of babies with Retinopathy of Prematurity (ROP) has increased (Royal College of Ophthalmologists (RCO), 2008). This presents a real challenge for neonatal nurses since their role in the screening programme is crucially important for early identification and appropriate treatment of this disease (RCO, 1995). Overall, the contribution of neonatal nurses to the national screening programme for congenital ophthalmic diseases is a significant issue that will be discussed in more detail in Chapter 8 of this book.

Engagement with technological advance has also been providing exciting opportunities for ophthalmic practitioners to extend their role and advance clinical practice. A constantly increasing knowledge and skills base has been manifesting itself effectively in the growing number of nurse-led approaches to diagnostic and measuring techniques, screening procedures, and minor surgery within ophthalmic practice. Substantial development has taken place in the areas of tonometry, biometry, intravenous fluorescein angiography, screening for diabetic retinopathy and glaucoma, photodynamic therapy and intravitreal therapy for the treatment of age-related macular degeneration

(AMD), and in minor surgical procedures such as removal of chalazion. Practitioners have also begun to apply their knowledge and understanding to the skills of undertaking HRT (Heidelberg Retinal Tomography) and OCT (Optical Coherence Tomography).

Intravenous fluorescein angiography

Undertaking fluorescein angiography is no longer the sole preserve of doctors. Senior ophthalmic practitioners are currently developing this procedure as a nurse-led approach. The scope of clinical practice for ophthalmic nurses in the outpatient clinic is gradually being extended, enabling them to perform peripheral venous cannulation for patients undergoing this procedure (Watkinson and Scott, 2003). The outcome of this innovative approach is that it has made a difference to the service offered in the outpatient clinic. It has given doctors more time to see more patients. In turn, this has reduced clinic overload and waiting lists, and helped nurses to meet their targets (Watkinson and Scott, 2003).

Diabetic retinal screening

Diabetic retinopathy poses a major challenge for the future in terms of an effective prevention strategy and appropriate care service provision. Ophthalmic nurse practitioners have already begun to respond to this enormous challenge by demonstrating their increased knowledge and skills in using appropriate technical equipment to perform retinal screening procedures such as slit-lamp bio-microscopy and digital photography. However, the challenge for the future is to develop their interpretative and diagnostic skills (Watkinson and Chetram, 2005). This requires the ability to recognise and interpret the stages of diabetic retinopathy, and the digital images of pathological retinal changes, alongside other significant ocular conditions such as cataract and glaucoma. Appropriate referrals for laser treatment can then be made (Watkinson and Chetram, 2005).

Photodynamic and intravitreal therapy

With advances in technology and drug therapy, the availability of photodynamic therapy (PDT) within the NHS has presented practitioners with a real opportunity to make a significant impact on the treatment of age-related macular degeneration (AMD).

Visudyne (verteporfin) therapy has become a recognised treatment for the wet (neovascular) form of AMD. Its distinct advantage is that it uses a combination of a photosensitive (light-activated) drug (verteporfin) and red light from a non-thermal laser (a laser that does not burn the retina). Indeed, NICE (2003) recommended the use of verteporfin PDT for selected patients whose vision was failing because of wet AMD. The available research evidence also suggested the value of its use in improving the chances of avoiding appreciable loss of vision over a period of two years (TAP Study Group, 2002). This treatment, however, is not suitable for all types of lesions and has recently been superseded by the advent of adjuvant therapies (Anti-VEGF) (Chong, 2006). These drugs are administered intravitreally and specifically bind to and inhibit the vascular endothelial growth factor (VEGF). The latter is a potent inducer of vascular permeability, stimulates angiogenesis, and may have pro-inflammatory effects, all of which are thought to contribute to the progression of neovascular AMD (Witmer et al., 2003). The current debate surrounding the two main anti-VEGF drugs in use, ranibizumab (Lucentis) and bevacizumab (Avastin), continues to be fuelled by research evidence emerging from ongoing randomised controlled trials as part of the government's drive for modelling the cost-effectiveness of such treatment (Moreno and Paloma, 2008; Rafferty et al., 2007).

Currently, NICE (2003) guidelines recommend that patients be fast-tracked to a treating retinal specialist within two weeks of suspecting wet AMD. Hopefully, this guideline will provide a basis for securing an effective service implementation. The ever-increasing ageing population has resulted in a greater demand for ophthalmic services, especially for the time and skills of the consultant retinal specialist. This demands a more efficient and effective use of resources. In turn, practitioners will be required to utilise their advanced knowledge and skills to become actively engaged in screening individuals referred with wet AMD, or suspected wet AMD. Ensuring that patients receive prompt, accurate diagnosis and appropriate treatment will perhaps be the overarching challenge. Alongside this, the key target for ophthalmic practitioners will be the effective management of newly referred patients requiring assessment.

Biometry and phakoemulsification

Overall, advanced surgical techniques have resulted in high-powered faster approaches such as phakoemulsification of lens, which removes a cataract speedily and effectively. Technical advances have been made in the product design of intra-ocular lenses. For example, intra-ocular lens (IOL) edge design now helps to reduce capsulotomy rates at one year. This is due to the square edge component of the lens, which serves as a barrier to migration of lens epithelial cells. Clearly, however, the success of such surgical techniques is dependent on precise anatomical measurement achieved through biometry. Correct IOL placement by the surgeon is vital, but using the correct IOL calculation formula is equally important. Thus, through the skill and accuracy required to perform such techniques, ophthalmic nurses make an essential contribution to successful surgical outcomes.

Ocular disease in the UK

Ocular disease in UK

In the UK, diseases such as diabetic retinopathy, age-related macular degeneration, and glaucoma are targeted as priority diseases.

Age-related macular degeneration

This is the most common disorder in the group of non-avoidable causes of visual loss. It is a painless disease of the macular area, most often clinically apparent after the age of 50 years (Kanski, 2007). It is a progressive degeneration of the macula in which the cells break down causing loss of sight in the central part of the field of vision, but leaving the peripheral or side vision unaffected. In the United Kingdom, it is the leading cause of visual impairment in people over the age of 65. Owen *et al.* (2003) estimate that there are currently 214,000 people in the UK with visual impairment caused by this condition. The number is expected to increase to 239,000 by the year 2011. Recent research evidence and the fact that there is no cure for AMD pose significant challenges for the professional practitioner for the future. The aim is to halt the disease process and arrest its progress. Although the cause of AMD is not fully understood, a combination of pre-disposing factors are thought to be responsible. These are age, diet and nutrition, sunlight, hypertension, raised cholesterol, genetics, smoking and gender. Health education will be essential in contributing to an overall prevention strategy. Several epidemiological surveys have demonstrated that smoking is a risk factor for AMD (Yorston, 2006). Smoking one pack of cigarettes per day for 40 years is associated with a three-fold increase in the risk of AMD (Yorston, 2006).Even passive smoking is associated with an increased risk, but stopping smoking appears to reduce the danger. Possibly 15 per cent of AMD cases are caused by smoking (Yorston, 2006). Diet and nutrition play an important role in AMD. Earlier epidemiological studies confirmed the benefits of a diet rich in carotenoids (antioxidants) in lowering the risk of this condition. However, current research suggests that there is insufficient evidence to support the role of dietary antioxidants, including the use of dietary antioxidant supplements, for the primary prevention of early AMD (Chong *et al.*, 2007). Excessive sun exposure has been proposed as a risk factor, but, again, not supported by published research studies (Khan *et al.*, 2006).

The major challenges for ophthalmic practitioners are to facilitate the diagnosis, management and ongoing treatment of patients (Watkinson and Scott, 2007). The use of effective counselling and health education skills will also help patients to move on emotionally (Watkinson and Scott, 2007). Patients with 'wet' AMD are twice as likely as other people in the population who have no sight-threatening problems to suffer depression and emotional distress (Blyth, 2006) and studies have shown that the average quality of life declines as a function of binocular visual loss (Brown *et al.*, 2000). How patients respond in their mind to their sight loss challenge is essential to their future well being. The longer-term aims are first to help patients to adjust to their visual loss, and second to promote their independence for self-management leading to the maintenance of vision and quality of lifestyle (Watkinson and Scott, 2007).

Glaucoma

The two main types of glaucoma occurring in adults are both sight threatening due to resulting optic nerve damage and therefore challenging in terms of their detection, treatment, and ongoing management. Acute closed angle glaucoma is an ocular emergency of sudden onset and must be treated immediately to avert an irreversible loss of sight. Initially, intensive medical treatment is given to reduce the intra-ocular pressure. Definitive treatment is surgery via a laser peripheral iridotomy, or surgical peripheral iridectomy to both eyes to prevent an attack occurring in the unaffected eye. Primary open angle glaucoma (POAG) has a non-dramatic onset, but is nevertheless one of the leading causes of blindness worldwide (Kass *et al.*, 2002). Individuals are at an increased risk of developing this condition because of elevated intra-ocular pressure or ocular hypertension (Kass *et al.*, 2002). Individuals with an intra-ocular pressure of between 24 and 32mmHg should be identified and assessed for the risk of developing POAG since they are more likely to benefit from early treatment (Kass *et al.*, 2002). Concordance with ocular hypotensive treatment is vital in reducing IOP as a means of preventing major sight loss. The future challenge for the nurse practitioner is to provide patient education for self-management and control of the condition. The most sobering issue is that there is no cure for POAG and the challenge for the ophthalmic nurse practitioner is to prevent a total loss of sight. Significantly, nurse-led initiatives in this area have resulted in the setting up of nurse-led glaucoma clinics and contributed to the development of patient education. The setting up of patient support groups has also played an important role in educating patients about the condition.

After AMD, glaucoma is one of the principal reasons for people needing to register as blind. Relatives should therefore also be made aware of the need for regular sight tests every two to three years since there is an increased familial risk of developing this condition. Eye tests are free for relatives of people with glaucoma aged 50 years and over (RNIB, 2004). Currently, people have to pay for their glaucoma eye medication, but this issue has considerable implications for those individuals who are in a disadvantaged financial position and simply not able to support such ongoing costs. The future challenge might well be how to prevent the compromise of eye health through uncontrolled IOP and gradual loss of sight and independence, and quality of life.

Diabetic retinopathy

Diabetic retinopathy (DR) is presenting a major challenge for all nurse practitioners worldwide for the twenty-first century. This is due in part to the predicted increase in the incidence of diabetes and its complications, of which diabetic retinopathy is one of the most devastating in terms of the ongoing retinal damage and gradual loss of sight. DR is a vascular complication of diabetes mellitus in which the small retinal blood vessels tend to degenerate after some years. Its incidence is primarily related to duration and control of the diabetes (Kanski, 2007). It is estimated that in 2002 diabetic retinopathy accounted for about 5% of world blindness, representing approximately 5 million blind people (WHO, 2008).

Diabetes mellitus is one of the commonest of all chronic medical conditions and represents a huge potential problem and one of the greatest challenges for the health services in the UK (NICE, 2008). There are currently over 2.5 million people with this condition and there are more than half a million people with undiagnosed diabetes (Diabetes, UK, 2008). Over 90% of people with diabetes have Type 2 (NICE, 2008). Current prevalence of Type 2 diabetes however is unknown and will vary with factors such as mix of ethnic groups and degree of social deprivation (NICE, 2008). In any case, current prevalence estimates are a poor pointer to the future burden of diabetes due to their continuing increase (NICE, 2008).

Diabetic retinopathy is the leading cause of blindness in people under the age of 60 in industrialised countries (NICE, 2002). Ninety per cent of people with Type 1 diabetes have some degree of diabetic retinopathy within 20 years of diagnosis and more than 60 per cent of people with type 2 diabetes will have this complication (NICE, 2004). In 2003 the government prioritised the screening of retinopathy in the UK as one of two critical national targets (DoH, 2003). By the end of 2006 it required a minimum of 80% of people with diabetes to be offered screening for the early detection and treatment of diabetic retinopathy rising to 100% by the end of 2007. Latest statistics suggest that three-quarters of a million people in England remain at risk of losing their sight because they are not being screened for diabetic retinopathy (Diabetes UK, 2008). Indeed, Diabetes UK is now calling for everyone aged 12 and over, diagnosed with diabetes, to have free digital retinal screening every year. This situation poses an enormous future challenge for ophthalmic practitioners in the UK. Currently, attempts are being made to meet this challenge by providing and developing nurse-led approaches to diabetes retinal screening. In doing this, a vitally important contribution is being made to the national screening programme for diabetics at risk of developing diabetic retinopathy (Watkinson and Chetram, 2005). Furthermore, their future role will be significant in providing effective evidence-based care as a basis for preventing blindness and maximising long-term quality of life for patients with diabetic retinopathy. The risk of visual impairment and blindness is substantially reduced by a care programme that combines methods for early detection with effective treatment of the diabetic retinopathy (NICE, 2002). Screening and treatment for diabetic retinopathy will not eliminate all cases of sight loss, but can play an important part in minimising the number of patients with sight loss due to retinopathy. Treatment options include laser photocoagulation for focal and diffuse maculopathy, and proliferative retinopathy. Maculopathy is the major cause of visual loss for people with Type 2 diabetes. Vitrectomy is performed for persistent vitreous haemorrhage and tractional retinal detachment involving the macula.

Although these treatment strategies are successful, older people need to be made aware of a number of risk factors as part of a preventative programme. Health education is clearly another important current and future challenge for ophthalmic practitioners. Older patients and their families will require reliable evidence and advice about the need to maintain good blood glucose and blood pressure control. Tight blood glucose and blood pressure control remains the cornerstone in the primary prevention of diabetic retinopathy (Mohamed et al., 2007). Good blood glucose control means maintaining levels at below HbA1c 6.5–7.5 per cent, depending on the individual's risk of macrovascular and microvascular complications (NICE, 2008). Maintaining good blood pressure is also important. If eye damage is already present, it is recommended the blood pressure be maintained at or below 130/80mmHg. Where no eye damage is present, an ideal target is at or below 140/80mmHg (NICE, 2008). Tight control of the blood pressure is a major modifiable factor for the incidence and progression of diabetic retinopathy (Mohamed *et al.*, 2007). Concordance with anti-hypertensive treatment is essential as patients with hypertension have a worse visual prognosis (UK Prospective Diabetes Study Group (UKPDS), 2004). Similarly, concordance with drug treatment to lower serum cholesterol levels is essential to reduce the incidence, rate of progression, and severity of diabetic retinopathy resulting in decreased visual acuity (The Eye Diseases Prevalence Research Group (EDPRG), 2004). Encouraging the regular checking of visual acuity to assess the onset of any severe pathological changes in the retina, and encouraging patients to keep their future hospital appointments, are also part of the nurse's role as a health educator.

Cataract

Cataract is a loss of transparency of the lens, which becomes opaque and impedes the light entering the eye. The condition causes a gradual loss of vision and eventually blindness, which is largely curable. Although most cataracts are related to ageing, occasionally children can be born with this condition, or a cataract may develop after eye injuries, inflammation, and other eye diseases. Cataract can be treated successfully by surgery to remove the opaque lens and replace it with an artificial plastic intraocular lens to restore sight. The incidence of cataract will inevitably increase with a growing older population, and it is an important cause of low vision in both developed and developing countries.

In the UK, cataract surgery has been transformed by an increased use of local anaesthesia, day-case surgery and phakoemulsification. However, the current problem is that the demand for cataract surgery in the UK exceeds its availability, and the best way to meet the demand remains a little unclear. A study by Tey *et al.* (2007) reports that a reorganisation of their existing National Health Service ophthalmic service increased the quality and volume of cataract surgery. It has been suggested that it would be advantageous for hospital cataract services to have an in-house treatment centre, where only cataract operations are performed. It is argued this model has improved the efficiency and quality of care and increased training opportunities for junior ophthalmologists. Other advantages of this model are that it is cost-effective, increases throughput, and is fully integrated with the local service (Tey *et al.*, 2007). During the past three years the number of people having cataract surgery has stabilised in England and Wales and waiting times have shortened with median waiting times at around 70 days (Wood, 2007). Currently, 95% of UK cataract procedures are still performed in NHS hospitals, but there might be a case for arguing that more procedures be performed in treatment centres.

Clearly, the argument for day-case surgery is overwhelming, but there is also current debate as to whether co-management would be a more advantageous option. This would involve delegating post-operative care to community optometrists. Practitioners in the day-care surgery setting face many challenges due to increasing workloads, but it might be argued that the delegation of such care would pose an even greater challenge. The current issues and challenges facing ophthalmic practitioners within the day-care cataract service are explored in more detail in Chapter 2.

Visual impairment and blindness in children

In the UK, an increase in ethnic diversity and greater survival of low birth weight babies is contributing to a higher proportion of children becoming visually impaired or blind (Rahi and Cable, 2003). This study also highlights how childhood visual impairment is associated with lower socio-economic status. Clearly, the role of the ophthalmic practitioner in screening and surveillance of ophthalmic disorders will be paramount for the future. The National Screening Committee (2006), having reviewed screening for ophthalmic disorders and visual defects in children, recommends that all children should be screened for visual impairment between four and five years of age. This should either be conducted by orthoptists or by professionals trained and supported by orthoptists.

Refractive error and low vision

Refractive errors include myopia (short-sightedness), and hyperopia (long-sightedness) with or without astigmatism. The magnitude of the problem poses a major challenge for ophthalmic practitioners and optometrists worldwide. Severe refractive errors have been estimated to account for about 5 million blind people. There are an estimated 124 million people in the world with low vision (WHO, 2008). The biggest challenge facing practitioners is the prevention and treatment of refractive errors through effective health education. Refractive errors can be rectified with appropriate optical correction and low vision may be helped with low vision devices.

Care and service provision

Care and provision

The impact of visual impairment on the provision of healthcare services for the future will be considerable. As already highlighted, with predicted growth of the older population, the incidence of visual impairment will increase significantly. One of the most important challenges for professional practitioners in ophthalmic and general practice will be trying to deliver quality care within the remit of cost-effective and efficient service provision.

Currently, the NHS and local authorities spend almost £20 billion on long-term and residential care, and nursing homes to support older people with visual impairment (DoH, 2001). Helping such people to maintain independence in their own homes would be much more cost-effective and reduce the burden of failing sight on the health services for the future. Again, the NHS spends £1.7 billion annually on treating hip fractures resulting from falls, mainly in older people whose failing eyesight has often been a contributory factor (DoH, 2001). Indeed, Legood et al. (2002) discovered that older people with sight problems are seven times more likely to fall and sustain a serious injury. Providing rehabilitation and mobility training to reduce the risk of falls could significantly reduce costs. Combining the treatment of poor vision with exercise and hazard management in the home has already produced an additional 14% reduction in the annual fall rate (Day et al., 2002). Thus, professional practitioners should be aware of the importance of regular eye examinations for older people and provide them with necessary advice, encouragement and support to undergo them. Certainly, one of the priorities of the government's National Service Framework (NSF) for Older People (DoH 2001) is to provide evidence-based specialist care to improve eye health screening and low vision services.

Other NSFs will also impact on the clinical practice of ophthalmic nurses for the future. The NSF for Diabetes sets out a ten-year programme of change to deliver world class care and support for people with diabetes, which also includes children and young people (DoH, 2003). It affirms that this can only be achieved through the development of clinical practice of nursing staff throughout the country (DoH, 2003).The main challenge is for practitioners to deliver better care to people with diabetes against the constraints of time. This means focusing on those patients who are at the greatest risk of developing the complications of diabetes, indicated by poor diabetes control, and those newly diagnosed with diabetes, where the opportunity to implement the NSF standards is greatest. Indeed, priorities for the NHS over the next three years are set out in the priorities and planning framework 2003–2006 (DoH, 2002). Significantly, for ophthalmic practitioners it established two critical targets for eye screening and the compilation of registers in the early stages of delivery. By the end of 2006, the government required a minimum of 80% of people with diabetes are to be offered screening for the early detection (and treatment, if needed) of diabetic retinopathy as part of a systematic programme that met national standards. This government target rose to 100% coverage of those at risk of retinopathy by the end of 2007.

Of particular importance to neonatal nurse practitioners is the NSF for children, young people, and maternity services (DoH, 2004). The main focus is on cultural change with reference to three targets: moving away from treating children as 'mini adults', promoting child and family-centred services, and focusing on providing age-appropriate care. Standard seven relates to hospital services. Recommendations made include minimising the time in hospital, providing daily access to a play specialist, and encouraging play techniques. Other key issues include offering choice over aspects of treatment or care, safety, well-being, careful history-taking, and appropriate reviews for child protection cases. Indeed, child protection issues are considered a priority within this framework. Safeguarding children and responding appropriately to signs and symptoms of abuse or neglect are highlighted (DoH, 2004). This is clearly a key area for all practitioners to address, but particularly for ophthalmic nurses. The detection of eye injuries or infections caused by physical or sexual abuse, or neglect will remain an ongoing challenge for the 21st century. This issue and its legal and ethical implications will be discussed in more detail in Chapter 8.

The future role of the ophthalmic practitioner

Future role of practitioner

Before reading on, I would like you to pause for thought and consider the following questions.

THINKING POINT 1

- Have you read the Darzi report (DoH, 2008) on the NHS in England?
- Are you excited by the proposals for the future role of the nurse?
- Are you ready to meet the NHS quality agenda for the 21st century?
- Are you ready as an ophthalmic practitioner to lead and make a difference?

The *High Quality Care for All* (DoH, 2008) report identifies four main themes, which include providing the most effective treatments, helping people to stay healthy, empowering patients, and keeping patients as safe as possible. These also represent the basis for the future role for ophthalmic nurse practitioners. Quality care is at the heart of the 21st century NHS agenda and is underpinned by the concepts of respect, personalised patient-centred care, care pathways, and patient autonomy (DoH, 2008). As Darzi points out, 'nurses will be at the heart of shaping patient experience and delivering care. Our ambition is to ensure that the NHS delivers high quality care in all aspects – an ambition that is impossible to achieve without high quality nursing' (DoH, 2008, p.17). He also suggests that it is important to continue to attract highly motivated and talented individuals, and to support nurses in leadership roles to achieve the required quality and excellence in care (DoH, 2008, p.17).

Clearly, high quality care is an important target for ophthalmic practitioners in all clinical settings, particularly in relation to older people. However the challenge is how high quality nursing can be achieved amidst the current local constraints within clinical practice such as bureaucracy, staff shortages, poor management and lack of leadership (DoH, 2008), which were identified earlier in this chapter. Undoubtedly, trying to manage these local issues presents some of the biggest challenges for ophthalmic practitioners for the 21st century. The Department of Health's Dignity in care initiative will be a significant future challenge for ophthalmic practitioners due to the increasing number of older people who, because of varying degrees of visual impairment, will require the respect, dignity, and privacy to maintain self-esteem, independence and quality of life (DoH, 2001).

In returning to a summary of the main issues discussed so far in this first chapter, it is clear that for the future, ophthalmic practitioners face many challenges in respect of the prevalence of ocular disease within the UK. The main challenges will be to provide health education, to maintain an updated knowledge of the main conditions giving rise to visual impairment, supported by current and appropriate research evidence, and to provide quality evidence-based care, advice and support. In the UK, health education, for example, plays a vitally important role in the prevention of eye injuries, which are a leading cause of visual impairment. As a current and future challenge it will be further discussed in Chapter 3, which examines the issues faced by ophthalmic practitioners in the accident and emergency department. Importantly, ophthalmic practitioners need to demonstrate competence. To this end the RCN Ophthalmic Nursing Forum (RCN, 2005) has provided a framework for use by practitioners in the context of a number of professional and political factors. Some of these include Agenda for Change (DoH, 1999), the need for leadership in specialist nursing, consistent provision of and access to ophthalmic nursing education throughout the UK, the need for work-based and lifelong learning, the NHS Plan (DoH, 2000), and National Service Frameworks and service modernisation. As the framework suggests, nurses are competent when they have the skills and abilities required for lawful, safe and effective professional practice without supervision (RCN, 2005).

Clearly, competence is also related to the ethical and legal issues surrounding the care and management of ophthalmic patients. Undoubtedly, these issues will challenge practitioners to maintain a robust approach to accountability within the growing complexities of professional practice and an increasingly litigious society. The NMC's (2008) recently updated Code of Practice has highlighted the areas of accountability, confidentiality, consent, management of risk and record keeping as being the cornerstone of fitness to practice. Implicit within this shared set of values is growing acknowledgement of patient rights and ethical practice. The overarching principles of the law and ethics and their application to ophthalmic practice, are given an in-depth discussion with specific examples from ophthalmic practice in Chapter 8 of this book. The issue of informed consent is discussed with specific reference to paediatric ophthalmic practice.

Importantly, the future role of ophthalmic practitioners and the advance of ophthalmic practice rest on a commitment to lifelong learning and professional knowledge development (Benner *et al.*, 1999). Advancing clinical practice will be achieved through developing the skills of reflection, critical appraisal of research evidence, and enhanced decision-making. Furthermore, the commitment to engage in research activities to promote a better understanding of the need for evidence-based practice will become the cornerstone of advanced ophthalmic practice and the advanced ophthalmic practitioner for the twenty-first century. These issues are given further consideration in the discussion in Chapter 10. The concept of the advanced ophthalmic practitioner receives more attention in Chapter 6 with specific reference to the ophthalmic theatre practitioner.

THINKING POINT 2

STOP AND PAUSE FOR THOUGHT AGAIN!

- How do you view ophthalmic practice for the future?
- How do you view yourself as an ophthalmic practitioner for the future?
- How can you change the 'culture' of ophthalmic practice?

From Figure 1.1, choose which emoticon summarises how you are feeling about the future right now. Make a note of this in your diary and compare it with how you feel when you reach the end of this book.

Figure 1.1   **Emoticons**

Conclusion

This first chapter has hopefully presented some food for thought in its overview of the most significant current issues and future challenges, alongside the local constraints, facing ophthalmic practitioners for the twenty-first century. The contributors of subsequent chapters within this book similarly adopt an interactive approach with the reader by the use of Thinking Points to stimulate critical thinking and problem-solving around further in-depth discussion of the issues and future challenges thus far presented.

References

Benner, P., Hooper-Kyriakidis, P., and Stannard, D. (1999). *Clinical Wisdom: Interventions in critical care – a thinking in action approach*. Philadelphia: WB Saunders.

Blyth, C. (2006). 'Developments for MD patients – a clinician's update.' *Digest. Journal of the Macular Disease Society* 61–4.

Brown, G. C., Sharma, S., Brown, M. M., and Kistler, J. (2000). 'Utility values and age-related macular degeneration,' *Archives of Ophthalmology* 118: 47–51.

Chong, E., Wong, T., Kreis, A., Simpson, J., and Guymer, R. (2007). 'Dietary antioxidants and primary prevention of age-related macular degeneration: systematic review and meta analysis.' *British Medical Journal* 355 (7623): 755.

Chong, V. (2006). 'Eye injection and AMD.' *Digest. Journal of the Macular Disease Society*, 65–9.

Day, L., Filders, B.. and Gordon, I. (2002). 'Randomised factorial trial of falls prevention among older people living in their own homes.' *British Medical Journal* 325 (7356): 128.

Department of Health (1999). *Making A Difference*. London: DoH.

Department of Health (1999). *Agenda for Change: modernising the NHS pay system*. London: DoH.

Department of Health (2000). *The NHS Plan: A Plan for Investment, A Plan for Reform*. London: The Stationery Office.

Department of Health (2001). *National Service Framework for Older People*. London: The Stationery Office.

Department of Health (2002). *Improvement, expansion and reform – the next 3 years: priorities and planning framework 2003–2006.*. London: DoH. www.dh.gov.uk/en/PublicationsandstatisticsPublications/PublicationsPolicyAnd Guidance/DH (accessed 20.5.09).

Department of Health (2003). *National Service Framework for Diabetes: Delivery Strategy*. London: DoH.

Department of Health (2004). *National Service Framework for Children, Young People and Maternity Services: Core standards*. London: DoH.

Department of Health (2008). *High Quality Care for All: NHS Next Stage Review final report*. London: DoH.

Diabetes UK (2008). *Guide to Diabetes*. London: Diabetes UK. www.diabetes.org.uk/Guide-to-diabetes/ (last accessed 20.10.08).

Eye Diseases Prevalence Research Group (2004). 'The prevalence of Diabetic Retinopathy among adults in the United States.' Archives of Ophthalmology 122: 552–63.

Kanski, J. (2007). *Clinical Ophthalmology*. Oxford: Blackwell.

Kass, M., Heuer, D., Higginbotham, E., Johnson, C., Keltner, J., Miller, J., Parrish, R., Wilson, M., and Gordon, M. (2002). 'The Ocular Hypertension Treatment Study: a randomized trial determines that topical ocular hypotensive medication delays or prevents the onset of primary open-angle glaucoma.' *Archives of Ophthalmology* 120 (6): 701–13.

Khan, J., Shahid, H., Thurlby, D., Bradley, M., Clayton, D., Moore, A., Bird, A., and Yates, J. (2006). 'Age-related macular degeneration and sun exposure, iris colour, and skin sensitivity to sunlight.' *British Journal of Ophthalmology* 90 (27): 39–40.

Legood, R., Scuffham, P., and Cryer, C. (2002). 'Are we blind to injuries in the visually impaired?' *Injury Prevention* 8 (2): 155–60.

Mohamed, Q., Gillies, M., and Wong, T.Y. (2007). 'Management of Diabetic Retinopathy: A systematic review.' *JAMA* 298 (8): 902–16.

Moreno, S.F., and Paloma, J.B. (2008). 'Therapeutic anti-VEGF in age-related macular degeneration: Ranibizumab and Bevacizumab controversy.' *British Journal of Ophthalmology* 92 (6): 866–7.

National Institute for Clinical Excellence (2002). Management of Type 2 Diabetes Retinopathy: Early Management and Screening. Available at www.nice.org.uk/pageaspx?o = 27915 (last accessed 16 February 2009).

National Institute of Clinical Excellence (2003). *Technology Appraisal Guidance 68. Guidance on the use of photodynamic therapy for age-related macular degeneration.* Available at www.nice.org.uk/Guidance/TA68/Guidance/pdf/English (last accessed 16 February 2009).

National Institute of Clinical Excellence (2004). *Falls. Assessment and Prevention of Falls in Older People. Clinical Guideline 2.* Available at: www.nice.org.uk/nicemedia/pdf/CG021NICEguideline.pdf (last accessed 16 February 2009).

National Institute of Clinical Excellence (2008). *Type 2 diabetes: the management of type 2 Diabetes. Clinical guideline 66.* Available at: www.nice.org.uk/nicemedia/pdf/CG066NICEGuidelineCorrectedDec08.pdf (last accessed 16 February 2009).

National Screening Committee (2006). *National Screening Committee Policy – vision defect screening (in children).* London: National Screening Committee, UK. Available at: www.library.nhs.uk/Eyes/ViewResource.aspx?resID = 60336 (last accessed 04/06/2008).

Nursing and Midwifery Council (2008). *The Code Standards of Conduct, Performance and Ethics for Nurses and Midwives.* London: Nursing and Midwifery Council.

Office for National Statistics (2008). *Census 2001: Population.* London: Office for National Statistics. Available at www.statistics.gov.uk/cci/nugget.asp?id = 185 (last accessed 30.11.08)

Owen, C., Fletcher, A., Donoghue, M., and Rudnika, A. (2003). 'How big is the burden of visual loss caused by age-related macular degeneration in the United Kingdom?' *British Journal of Ophthalmology* 87 (3): 312–17.

Rafferty, J., Clegg, A., Jones, J., Tan, S.C., and Lotery, A. (2007). 'Ranibizumab (Lucentis) versus bevacizumab (Avastin): modelling cost-effectiveness.' *British Journal of Ophthalmology* 91: 1244–6.

Rahi, J., and Cable, N. (2003). 'Severe visual impairment and blindness in children in the UK. British Childhood Visual Impairment Study Group.' *The Lancet* 362 (9393): 1359–65.

Royal College of Nursing (2005). *Competencies: An Integrated Career and Competency Framework for Ophthalmic Nursing.* London: RCN.

Royal College of Ophthalmologists & British Association of Perinatal Medicine (1995). *Retinopathy of Prematurity Guideline for the Screening and Treatment.* The Report of a Joint Working Party. London: RCOP.

Royal College of Ophthalmologists (2008). *UK Retinopathy of Prematurity Guideline for the Screening and Treatment of Retinopathy of Prematurity.* London: RCO.

Royal National Institute of the Blind (2004). *Understanding Glaucoma.*
Available at: www.rnib.org.uk/xpedio/groups/public/documents/publicwebsite/
public_rnib003655.hcsp#P112_10351 (last accessed 12 May 2008).

Tey, A., Grant, B., Harbison, D., Sutherland, S., Kearns, P., and Sanders, R.
(2007). 'Redesign and modernisation of an NHS cataract service (Fife
1997–2004): multifaceted approach.' *British Medical Journal* 334: 148–52.

Treatment of Age-related Macular Degeneration with Photodynamic Therapy
(TAP) Study Group (2002). 'Verteporfin therapy for subfoveal choroidal neovas-
cularization in age-related macular degeneration. Three-year results of an open-
label extension of 2 randomized clinical trials – TAP Report No. 5.' *Archives of
Ophthalmology* 120: 1307–14.

UK Prospective Diabetes Study (UKPDS) Group (2004). 'Risks of progression of
retinopathy and vision loss related to tight blood pressure control in Type 2
Diabetes Mellitus.' *Archives of Ophthalmology* 122: 1631–40.

United Nations Population Division (UNPD) (2002). *World Population Prospects:
The 2000 Revision, Volume 3: Analytical Report.* New York: United Nations.

Watkinson, S., and Chetram, N. (2005). 'A nurse-led approach to diabetic
retinal screening.' *Nursing Times* 101 (36): 32–4.

Watkinson, S., and Scott, E. (2003). 'Nurse-led management of IV fluorescein
angiography.' *Nursing Times* 99 (18): 34–5.

Watkinson, S., and Scott, E. (2007). 'The role of the ophthalmic nurse specialist
in enhancing the care and management of patients undergoing photodynamic
therapy.' *Journal of European Society of Nurses and Technicians* 1 (3): 27–35.

Witmer, A., Vrenson, G., Van Noorden, C., and Schlingemann, R. (2003).
'Vascular endothelial growth factors and angiogenesis in eye disease.' *Progress
in Retinal and Eye Research* 22: 1–29.

Wood, C. (2007). 'Surgery for cataract.' *British Medical Journal* 334 (7585): 107.

World Health Organization (1999). *Vision 2020: the Right to Sight.* Geneva:
WHO.

World Health Organization (2008). *Priority Eye Diseases.* Geneva: WHO.
Available at: www.who.int/blindness/causes/priority/en/index5.html
(last accessed 2 June 2008).

Yorston, D. (2006). 'What's new in age-related macular degeneration?'
Community Eye Health Journal 19 (57): 4–5.

Chapter 2

Pre-assessment of day-case cataract surgery

Anthony Afanu

Objectives of pre-operative assessment
The role of the nurse in pre-assessment clinic
Cancellation of surgery
Patient group directions
Telephone pre-assessment
One-stop cataract surgery

Introduction

Chapter 1 presented an overview of some of the issues and challenges facing current and future ophthalmic practice. It also discussed the impact of demographic changes, technological advances, government initiatives, and the increased demand for cataract surgery as some of the issues facing healthcare professionals involved in the provision of day-case cataract surgery. In England, for example, government policies and initiatives such as the Department of Health's Action on Cataracts (2000), and NHS Improvement Plan (2004) require healthcare institutions to reduce waiting times for cataract surgery as well as deliver quality healthcare to patients. This situation exerts considerable pressure on healthcare professionals as they are expected to deliver quality care, meet organisational targets and also cope with increasing workload due to demographic changes as explained in Chapter 1. Clearly, healthcare professionals involved in the provision of day-case surgery should have the ability to work under pressure as well as deliver safe, effective and efficient service. However, the pace of modern day-case surgery means that thorough and accurate pre-operative assessment is essential for the provision of quality day surgery.

This chapter therefore aims to explore and discuss further some of the important issues and challenges of current and future ophthalmic practice but with particular attention to pre-assessment of day-case cataract surgery. Pre-operative assessment is seen as a process to ensure patients are fit for surgery, anaesthetic, understand the proposed operation and are ready to proceed (NHS Modernisation Agency, 2002a). But, almost half of day surgery patients are not pre-assessed for suitability before they arrive for their operation and, many other day surgery units also acknowledge pre-assessing only selected patients before day of surgery (Healthcare Commission, 2005). This situation is worrying as it increases the risk of cancellation of operation on the day of surgery, delays and long hours of waiting for patients to undergo surgery and discharge, which can be inconveniencing and frustrating.

In the UK, cataract care has undergone service modernisation following the publication of Department of Health's Action on Cataracts (NHS Executive, 2000), and the Royal College of Ophthalmologists Cataract Surgery Guidelines (2004). As a result, day-case rate for cataract surgery has increased from 88 per cent in 2000/2001, to 96 per cent in 2006/2007 (NHS Institute for Innovation and Improvement, 2008). It is therefore expedient that healthcare organisations adopt a sound pre-assessment process and guidelines essential to determine patient suitability for day surgery, enhance efficient use of day surgery services, provide high quality healthcare, and positive patient experience. It is with these views that this chapter aims to discuss the objectives of pre-operative assessment, the role of the nurse in pre-assessment clinics, cancellation of surgery, patient group directions, telephone pre-assessment, and one-stop cataract surgery as some of the important issues and challenges of pre-operative assessment of day-case cataract surgery.

Objectives of pre-operative assessment

Objectives of assessment

Adequate preparation is vital for any successful day-case cataract surgery. Preparation starts as soon as the decision to operate is made, and during pre-operative assessment of patients. In healthcare settings, assessment involves gathering of information and formulation of judgements regarding a person's health situation, needs and wishes, which should guide further action (Heath, 2000). Pre-operative assessment of patients scheduled for day-case cataract surgery should therefore be geared towards determining their suitability for anaesthetic and surgery, improving their understanding of proposed surgery, ensuring safe performance and outcome of surgery (RCOA and RCOph, 2001).

The main objective of pre-operative assessment is to ensure patients are fit for surgery, and a care plan put in place to ensure improved surgical outcome (RCOph, 2004). Walsgrove (2006) summarises the main aims of pre-operative assessment as follows (see Box 2.1).

Box 2.1

Main aims of pre-operative assessment
Adapted from Walsgrove (2006)

- To minimise patient risk.
- To identify patient suitability and/or fitness for surgery/anaesthesia.
- To provide information for informed choices and consent.
- To reduce fears and anxieties.
- To assist better use of theatre and ward resources.
- To improve the surgical patient's hospital experience.

The role of the nurse in the pre-assessment clinic

Role of the nurse in pre-assessment

The role of the nurse in pre-operative assessment includes assessing, planning, and implementing measures necessary to ensure safe and effective delivery of healthcare that meets individual patient needs. Undoubtedly, this role is challenging as the nurse is expected to provide quality service as well as cope with increased workload, perform accurate biometry and slit lamp microscopy essential in contributing to successful surgical outcome. It is therefore important that trained ophthalmic nurses and cataract pre-operative assessment practitioners have a thorough working knowledge of patient assessment so that they can contribute to the provision of quality day-case cataract surgery.

Utilising an assessment tool based on a nursing care model is beneficial during assessment as it incorporates the plan of care for the day of surgery, and for discharge home. Theoretical nursing frameworks significantly influence modern practice, hence, ophthalmic units should endeavour to link theory to practice when developing their own criteria for assessing patient suitability for day-case cataract surgery. For example, Roper *et al.* (2000) focus on activities of daily living whilst Orem's (1995) self-care model places emphasis on self-care, autonomy and the promotion of patients' ability to meet their own care needs wherever possible. Clearly, the desired nursing outcome for pre-operative assessment of ophthalmic patients is to enhance their self-care at home as individuals or with assistance of carers (Stanford, 1998). The Royal College of Anaesthetists (2006) suggest that, best practice in pre-assessment clinics should include the following (see Box 2.2):

Box 2.2

Day surgery services:
best practice in pre-admission assessment
Adapted from: The Royal College of Anaesthetists (2006)

- Pre-assessment should be performed by trained nurses and supported by anaesthetists/surgeons (NHS Modernisation Agency, 2004).

- Pre-assessment process should be protocol-driven; structured questionnaires are useful in data collection (AAGBI, 2005).

- Assessment should be based on social and medical criteria, according to recent national good practice guidelines on pre-operative assessment and agreed with anaesthetic department (NHS Modernisation Agency 2002a).

- Assessment should be performed in time to correct any abnormalities and allow the patient to be adequately informed and prepared for surgery (NHS Modernisation Agency, 2004).

Anecdotal reports suggest that the role of the ophthalmic nurse in cataract pre-assessment clinics varies from one Trust to another depending on the needs of the institution and local protocols. The

Royal College of Anaesthetists and The Royal College of Ophthalmologists (2001) indicate that nurses generally undertake pre-operative assessment clinics but the final responsibility rests with the anaesthetist and surgeon. However, qualified ophthalmic nurses in pre-assessment clinics have the capability to perform the following roles (eye examination, special investigations, general health evaluation, communication, and patient education) safely and efficiently.

Eye examination

In cataract pre-assessment clinics, qualified ophthalmic nurses are faced with the challenge of performing accurate visual assessment essential to establish best-corrected visual acuity for distance, near vision, binocular vision and amblyopia. Other elements of ocular examination should include measurement of intraocular pressure, testing for relative afferent papillary defect, and slit lamp microscopy. A thorough eye examination is also important to assist diagnosis of visually significant cataract, exclude coexisting ocular disease (blepharitis, conjunctivitis, dry eyes, lacrimal dysfunction) and alert surgeons to potential areas of increased risk to cataract surgery (Allan, 2001). Patients with obscured fundus view should be referred to the ophthalmologist for further examination and special investigation, e.g. B-scan ultrasonography to establish whether the retina is attached and identify any intraocular lesions.

Special investigations

Biometry and keratometry: Performing accurate biometry and keratometry has increasingly become a challenge to pre-assessment ophthalmic practitioners, as it is an essential part of a successful cataract operation. Biometry and keratometry investigations are performed to establish the correct lens implant to use during cataract surgery that meets the refractive needs of an individual patient (NHS Executive, 2000). These special investigations require specialised skill but are very often underestimated. It is therefore expedient that suitably trained healthcare professionals (ophthalmic nurses, technicians, optometrists, orthoptists, and ophthalmologists) perform these investigations so as to obtain accurate readings.

These investigations should be performed in advance of surgery to allow time for the appropriate intraocular lens (IOL) to be ordered. According to the Royal College Ophthalmology (2004) there are two components of biometry investigation:

- Axial length (AL) measurement by A-scan ultrasound or laser interferometry and
- Corneal curvature (K1, K2) measurement by keratometry or corneal topography.

Both eyes should be measured even if unilateral surgery is planned to allow for crosschecking. Similarly, focimetry should be carried out or the latest copy of the patient's refraction cross-referenced with the biometry results, taking into account the effect of the cataract on refraction. It is important to keep biometry printouts in patients' notes with their names, hospital number and date of birth clearly marked on them. Biometry instruments should be serviced regularly, calibrated daily and operated in accordance with manufacturer's instruction manual to ensure effective functioning of equipment.

There are different formulae used in intraocular lens calculations for the selection of the correct lens implant to use during cataract surgery. SRK/T is regarded as a very good general formula (RCOph, 2004). It is important to check and use the appropriate formula and constants in order to prevent inaccurate results and IOL calculation. See Table 2.1 for a summary of axial length measurement and its recommended formula.

Table 2.1

Axial length measurement

Adapted from The Royal College of Ophthalmologists (2004)

Axial length (mm)	Formula
< 22mm	Hoffer Q or SRK/T
22–24.5mm	SRK/T or Holladay
> 24.6mm	SRK/T

The Royal College of Ophthalmologists (2004) also provides information on biometry data, which includes the following:

- 96 per cent of axial lengths fall within the range 21.0mm to 25.5mm and for 60 per cent of axial lengths, it is between 22.5 and 24.5mm.

- 98 per cent of K-readings fall within the range of 40 to 48D and 68 per cent of K-readings are between 42 and 45D.

- In the absence of pathology (e.g. unilateral refractive error, coloboma or staphyloma) that might affect eye size, most individuals have similar axial lengths in each eye.

- Most corneas are relatively regularly curved and similar between the two eyes of one individual.

- Any intraocular difference in axial length of more than 0.3mm or K readings which vary by more than one dioptre require confirmation. These results should only be accepted when repeated measurements show consistent results.

- When there are large differences between the K readings and/or axial lengths, consider the possibility of amblyopia or vitreous opacities such as asteroid hyalosis. Amblyopic eye may have been forgotten by the patient and may not be corrected in the current spectacle prescription.

- For highly myopic eyes (axial > 28mm) a B-scan should be carried out to determine the presence or otherwise of staphyloma.

General health evaluation

Practitioners should endeavour to undertake detailed medical and surgical history of patients scheduled for day-case cataract surgery to enable them to elicit medical, social, and psychological problems so as to determine patients' suitability for day surgery and anaesthetic. A good medical and surgical history is important to enable the practitioner to assess patients' ability to instil eye drops after discharge, maintain their own safe environment at home after general anaesthetic, and also establish their ability to cooperate and lie reasonably flat during the surgery. For instance, patients with severe Parkinson's disease may be considered for general anaesthetic whilst patients with hiatus hernia or chronic obstructive airways disease may need to have their head slightly raised during surgery.

General health evaluation should include blood pressure check to establish any high blood pressure (hypertension), record of allergies, note of current medications (warfarin, tamsulosin, and aspirin), and possibly investigations to include blood test, ECG, and X-ray if necessary.

Hypertension: All patients attending cataract pre-assessment clinics should have their blood pressure checked as part of their medical evaluation before the day of surgery. Patients found to have high blood pressure readings during pre-assessment clinics should be referred to their primary physician for pre-operative blood pressure control before surgery. The Royal College of Anaesthetists and the Royal College of Ophthalmologists (2001) define hypertension as a systolic arterial blood pressure (SBP) at or above 180 mm Hg or a diastolic arterial pressure (DBP) above 100 mmHg. They further suggest that rapid lowering of blood pressure immediately prior to surgery is not advisable and patients should continue to take their medications up to and including the day of surgery.

Anecdotal reports however show that strict adherence to systolic blood pressure at or above 180 mm Hg and diastolic blood pressure above 100 mm Hg on the day of surgery will result in a number of cancellations of patients presenting for cataract surgery. Anxiety and apprehension associated with 'white coat syndrome' can be a reason for increased blood pressure readings on the day of surgery. However, ensuring that patients are well-informed, offering explanation and opportunity for discussion and adequate psychosocial preparation pre-operatively can minimise anxiety and apprehension associated with day surgery (Mitchell, 2002).

It is therefore important to compare blood pressure readings during pre-operative assessment to readings on the day of surgery so as to make good clinical judgement on a patient's blood pressure status. Local protocols designed with measures to control raised blood pressure on the day of surgery should be utilised before patients are considered unsuitable for cataract operation.

Allergies: It is important to record all allergies and their adverse effects in patients' notes so as to ensure safe practice. For instance, patients allergic to sulphonamides should not be administered acetazolamide, which is sometimes administered to patients to prevent rise in intra-ocular pressure after cataract surgery. Some patients may also be allergic to penicillin or its derivatives, which are very often the drug of choice for sub-conjunctival injection at the end of cataract surgery (Stanford, 1998). In some cases, patients may not have drug allergies but may have adverse reaction to surgical tapes used to secure dressings after cataract surgery or react to latex surgical gloves used during cataract surgery. It is therefore important for pre-operative assessment ophthalmic practitioners to report appropriately any patient allergy so as to ensure no harm is done to the patient during or after cataract surgery.

Current medications

Warfarin: Warfarin is an oral anticoagulant commonly used in conditions where clotting could have severe or life-threatening consequences. Warfarin also has the tendency to cause sight-threatening haemorrhages in cataract surgery (Rotenstreich *et al.*, 2001). All patients on warfarin scheduled for cataract surgery should have the effect of their anticoagulation therapy checked the day before surgery to ensure INR (International Normalised Ratio) is within therapeutic range safe for surgery. The Royal College of Anaesthetists and Royal College of Ophthalmologists (2001) stress the importance of the patient's INR being known for procedures involving sharp needles or sub-Tenon's block due to the risk of bleeding.

According to Dewsbury (2003), the World Health Organisation's reference international sensitivity index (ISI) for warfarin is 1 (mean normal prothrombin time in seconds) and the standard INR range for most clinical situations is 2 to 3. However, in patients who have had recurrent thromboses or have heart prostheses, the INR may be 2.5 to 3.5. The Royal College of Anaesthetists and Royal College of Ophthalmologists (2001) recommend that INR should be within the therapeutic ratio, which should be determined by the condition for which the patient is being anticoagulated. It is therefore important for pre-assessment nurses or day surgery staff to discuss any high INR with the anti-coagulation service, surgeon, and anaesthetist so as to identify the required range and adjust warfarin to ensure INR level is safe for the patient and cataract surgery.

Hirschman and Morby (2006) report possible complications associated with anticoagulation therapy including:

- anaesthesia-related bleeding (bruising, sub-conjunctival haemorrhage, retrobulba, peribulba, and expulsive haemorrhage)

- intraocular surgery-related bleeding (choroidal or vitreous haemorrhage, hyphaema, retinal detachment, or expulsive haemorrhage).

However some studies indicate that continuation of anticoagulation therapy during cataract surgery does not significantly increase the risk of sight-threatening complications; instead discontinuation of warfarin or anticoagulation therapy pre-operatively does indeed risk life-threatening systemic complications such as death from cerebrovascular accident, transient ischaemic attack, myocardial infarction, and pulmonary embolism (Konstantos, 2001; Rotenstreich *et al.*, 2001; Hirschman and Morby, 2006). Pre-assessment and day surgery units should therefore consider a well-designed local protocol with input from the haematologists, anaesthetists, and surgeons with a view to consider the benefits of continuations of anticoagulation therapy in preventing thromboembolic events as against the discontinuation of warfarin to minimise sight-threatening complications.

The Royal College of Ophthalmology (2004) suggests the following for patients on warfarin scheduled for cataract surgery:

- The INR should be checked to ensure patients are within their desired therapeutic range set by the physician.
- Consideration should be given to using either sub-Tenon's or topical anaesthesia.
- If needle local anaesthesia is performed, the risk of orbital haemorrhage is increased by 0.2–1.0%.

Tamsulosin (Flomax): Tamsulosin is an alpha-blocker licensed for the treatment of benign prostatic hyperplasia (BPH). However, it blocks α-1A receptors of the iris dilator smooth muscle thereby increasing the risk of intraoperative floppy iris syndrome (IFIS) during cataract surgery (Chang and Campbell, 2005). Inadequate pupil dilation associated with patients taking tamsulosin is a potential source of surgical complication (posterior capsule rupture, and vitreous loss) during cataract surgery as the pupil immediately snaps back to its original size following any attempt to stretch it (Chang and Campbell, 2005; Vasavada and Singh, 2000).

Chang and Campbell (2005) report that tamsulosin has a long half-life of 48 to 72 hours and relatively constant blockage of α-1A receptors and therefore should temporarily be withdrawn two weeks before cataract surgery. MHRA (2006) however argues that tamsulosin is an irreversible antagonist of α-1A adrenoceptors, and thus a withdrawal period of several days may not be sufficient to suppress the blockage of α-1A adrenoceptors. The benefits of withdrawing tamsulosin therefore remain unclear even though discontinuation of one to two weeks before cataract surgery is anecdotally helpful (MHRA, 2006).

A good working knowledge of tamsulosin is therefore needed for cataract pre-assessment nurses to keep patients well-informed. Ophthalmic pre-assessment units should adopt local protocols to ensure patients who are or have been treated with tamsulosin are identified and surgeons appropriately notified prior to cataract surgery so as to minimise the complications associated with IFIS.

Aspirin: Aspirin is used for the prophylaxis of cerebro-vascular disease or myocardial infarction (BNF, 2007). Konstantos (2001) however argues that aspirin is little better than a placebo in the prevention of thrombotic events as compared to warfarin. A study on the effect of aspirin intake on bleeding during cataract surgery found little difference in intraoperative bleeding between patients taking aspirin and those who stopped 2 to 5 or 7 to 10 days before cataract surgery (Assia *et al.*, 1998). The inference, although not stated in any of these studies, appears to suggest that patients face no additional risk of sight-threatening bleeding with continuous intake of aspirin before cataract surgery. Besides, utilisation of topical and sub-Tenon's blocks for cataract surgery has helped to prevent any sight-threatening bleeding complication associated with continuous intake of aspirin before cataract surgery.

Investigations

Unless there is a specific clinical indication, blood test, ECG, and X-rays are not necessary before cataract surgery (NHS Executives, 2000). However, in some institutions, pre-assessment practitioners routinely perform standard investigations (blood test and ECG) for some categories of patients scheduled for cataract surgery requiring general anaesthesia.

Communication

Effective communication by pre-assessment practitioners with appropriate units during a patient's care journey is vital for successful day-case cataract surgery as it facilitates the provision of safe, effective, and efficient seamless service to patients. It is important for practitioners to communicate any special need or requirements identified during pre-operative assessment to the appropriate department so as to facilitate efficient use of theatre time and day surgery resources. For example, issues with lack of hearing and understanding of English may be challenging during general anaesthetic induction or local anaesthetic administration. As such, appropriate documentation of a patient's inability to hear or understand English and the necessary action to secure a link worker or interpreter at all stages of care is essential for effective care and efficient utilisation of day surgery resources. Patients with hearing aids should be encouraged to wear them to enhance hearing and understanding. However, if hearing aids are removed during cataract surgery to prevent them from being wet, care should be taken not to lose them.

It is important for each consultant list to have a designated pre-assessment practitioner to check results of patient investigations and ensure abnormal results are acted upon to avoid later cancellations. Besides, checking of operating lists and notes of patients at least one week prior to admission minimises last minute errors and consequential cancellations, as there is time to correct errors and inappropriate listing.

Patient education

The role of the ophthalmic nurse in patient education during pre-operative cataract assessment is important to keep patients well-informed, ehance their confidence and overall experience, ensure patients arrive on time and are adequately prepared to proceed with surgery. It is also important for ophthalmic practitioners to discuss admission requirements, time of arrival, fasting times, taking of medications, what to expect on the day of surgery, during the operation, and discharge information to include instructions on eye drops instillation and ocular hygiene. Practitioners should also discuss patients' concerns and their expectations, clarify any issue of uncertainty, offer patients the opportunity to ask questions and obtain patient confirmation to proceed with recommended surgery (NHS Modernisation Agency, 2002a). Patient education during the pre-operative assessment should include provision of information (verbal and written) to patients and their family to enhance their knowledge, compliance and ensure eye safety. However, ophthalmic practitioners should endeavour to establish what information patients need and balance that with what they wish to know in order to empower them to seek knowledge (Stanford, 1998). The purpose of patient education within the empowerment philosophy is to provide information that will help patients make informed decisions about their care, obtain clarity about their goals, values, motivation and assume responsibility for their own care (Funnell and Anderson, 2004). The provision of the desired level of information to patients during pre-operative assessment is also central in alleviating anxiety associated with day-case surgery (Mitchell, 1999).

Pre-operative information can be offered verbally and reinforced with written information leaflets, visual presentations, and a model of the eye or the use of audiovisual aids. It is also appropriate for ophthalmic practitioners in pre-operative assessment clinics to consider a strategic framework for patient education to achieve optimum eye health. For example, Tannahill and Downie's (1990) health promotion model incorporates the overlap of health education, health promotion and prevention. This could be utilised in patient education to teach patients effective hand washing before eye drop instillation, which contributes to prevention of infection and promotion of eye health.

THINKING POINT I

TAKE A FEW MINUTES AND REFLECT ON YOUR OWN PRACTICE AREA

- What criteria do you have for assessing patient suitability for day-case cataract surgery?
- What role(s) do your pre-assessment ophthalmic nurses play in ensuring patient suitability for day surgery?
- Reflect on your pre-assessment process and describe/outline how it contributes to positive day surgery experience.

Cancellation of surgery

About two-thirds of all cancelled operations in day surgery are cancelled by patients (NHS Modernisation Agency, 2002a) whilst 25 per cent of day surgery units also cancel more than 9 per cent of intended procedures (Healthcare Commission, 2005). This is a serious concern as it results in waste of resources for NHS organisations, and also is distressing and inconveniencing to patients. Cancelled operations whether by patients or NHS trust can be problematic for the hospital as it involves significant amounts of administrative work of re-scheduling appointments. Patients on the other hand also have the frustration and challenge of re-arranging their home circumstances to suit new appointments. It is therefore necessary for healthcare organisations to identify and understand the different types and reasons for cancellations (see Figure 2.1) so as to adopt appropriate measures to improve hospital efficiency and positive patient experience.

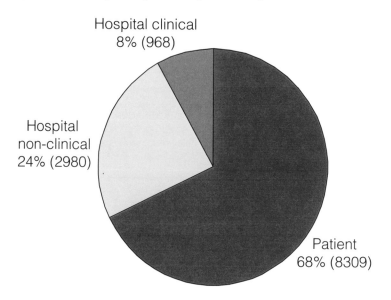

Figure 2.1

Source of all day case cancellations, Aug 01–Jun 02
Adapted from NHS Modernisation Agency (2002a).

The NHS Modernisation Agency (2002a) explains the three sources of day-case cancellations as follows:

- Hospital non-clinical cancellations (consultant unavailable, administrative error, emergencies, list over-run, equipment failure or unavailable, and theatre staff unavailable).

- Hospital clinical cancellations (operation not necessary, pre-operative assessment protocol not followed, patient arrived with illness and pre-existing medical condition).

- Patient cancellations (operation not required, unfit for surgery, appointment inconvenient, and 'did not attend's).

However, for pre-operative assessment to be effective in reducing the number of cancelled operations, it must be implemented in the context of a wider system including elective and emergency surgical admission, operating theatres, bed management, and discharge planning (NHS Modernisation Agency, 2002b).

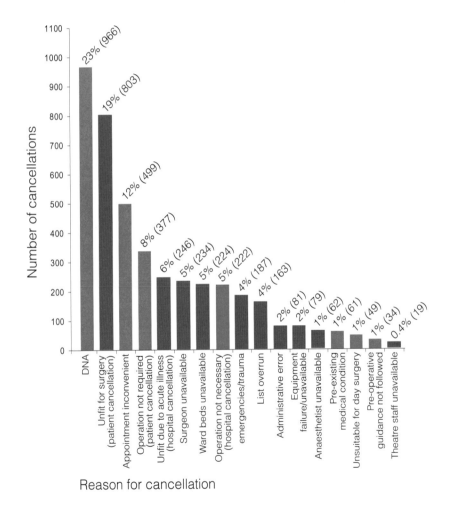

Figure 2.2

Reasons for day case cancellations, Aug 01–Jun 02
Adapted from NHS Modernisation Agency (2002a).

NHS Modernisation Agency (2002b) also suggests the following actions in tackling cancelled operations:

- tackling operating list overruns
- looking into consultant and theatre staff availability
- scheduling emergencies and trauma
- dealing with equipment failure and availability, and
- understanding and reducing patient cancellations
  (see Figure 2.2 on p. 37 for reasons of day-case cancellations).

Evidence from a pilot theatre programme in nine NHS trusts in England from August to June 2001 reveals that effective pre-operative assessment minimises the risk of late cancellations and also decreases the number of 'Did Not Attend's (NHS Modernisation Agency, 2002a). Also, sending text messages or making telephone calls to patients a week or two prior to their admission can also decrease the number of 'Did Not Attend's. Expanding pre-operative assessment to include more time for detailed discussion with patients about their surgery, noting requirement for admission, surgery and discharge, and facilitating patient choice of date can potentially prevent about half of all day surgery cancellations (NHS Modernisation Agency, 2002a).

Patient group directions

Patient group directions

Patient group direction (PGD) is a specific written instruction for the supply and administration of a named medicine in an identified clinical situation where the group of patients may not be individually identified before presenting for treatment (NMC, 2002). The desire for day surgery units to ensure patients are discharged early with their 'To Take Out or Home' (TTO) medications after surgery is a notable challenge as patients have to wait for considerable hours before their TTOs arrive from pharmacy. Such delays are worrying as it is often stressful and inconveniencing to patients and their relatives who are eager to return home without unnecessary delay in hospital. It is therefore expedient for healthcare organisations to organise and provide services around patient needs so as to deliver quality service that is patient-centred. Hence, there is a need for patient group directions to be utilised to prescribe, supply and administer specific medicines in accordance with appropriate professional organisational accountability.

Patient group directions would enable practitioners to supply TTOs from their unit as opposed to patients waiting for TTOs from pharmacy. Anecdotal reports suggest that patient group direction reduces waiting time for patients to collect their TTOs, minimises unnecessary delay and therefore enables early discharge of patients after day-case cataract surgery. PGD also minimises wastage associated with re-labelling of pre-ordered medications for patients cancelled on the day of surgery. Professional groups who can use patient group direction include: midwives, nurses, pharmacists, optometrists, podiatrists and chiropodists, radiographers, orthoptists, physiotherapists and ambulance paramedics (Picton *et al.*, 2004). Patient group directions, however, must clearly benefit patients, meet an identified clinical need, contribute to effective use of resources, and must not comprise patient safety or put them at risk (Dick, 2005). Clinical guidelines or consensus statements should underpin patient group directions and should include the following information (Picton *et al.*, 2004):

- the name of the body to which the direction applies
- the date the direction comes into force and the date it expires
- a description of the medicine(s) to which the direction applies
- the clinical conditions covered by the direction
- a description of those patients excluded from treatment under the direction
- a description of the circumstances under which further advice should be sought from a doctor, pharmacist, (or as appropriate) and arrangements for referral made
- appropriate dosage and maximum total dosage, quantity, prescription form and strength, route and frequency of administration, and minimum or maximum period over which the medicine should be administered
- relevant warnings, including potential adverse reactions
- details of any follow-up action and the circumstances, and
- a statement of the records to be kept for audit purposes.

Patient group directions should be authorised by the trust, specifically by the director of pharmaceutical services, the trust risk manager and the medical director and should be drawn up by a multidisciplinary group including a doctor, a pharmacist and a representative of each of the professions likely to work within the protocol (Dick, 2005).

THINKING POINT 2

TAKE FEW MINUTES AND REFLECT ON YOUR OWN PRACTICE AREA.

- What do you consider are some of the issues and challenges of pre-operative assessment of day-case cataract surgery within your clinical area?

- What are some of the innovations and initiatives within your clinical area that you consider are helping to manage some of these issues and challenges?

- Reflect on your clinical area and outline what promotes the delivery of high quality pre-operative assessment service to day-case cataract patients.

- How would you contribute to positive day surgery experience within your clinical area?

Telephone pre-assessment

Telephone pre-assessment

Recent increase in the number of patients scheduled for day surgery coupled with inadequate space and staffing has rendered the traditional face-to-face pre-assessment of patients before surgery challenging. Telephone pre-assessment is one of the ways of addressing this situation. Gaskell *et al.* (2001) emphasise the value of telephone pre-assessment as it reduces the need for patients to attend hospital for pre-operative assessment before surgery. Digner (2007) reports the benefits of telephone pre-assessment to include the following:

- Pre-operative assessments are completed at the convenience of patients in their homes and at a time that suits them.

- Patients do not have to attend hospital for a further visit prior to surgery as they previously did.

- Telephone pre-assessment reduces the need for patients to take more time off and struggle with car parking at the hospital.

- It improves theatre utilisation by reducing the rate of patients who did not attend day surgery units for surgery (DNAs).
- Telephone pre-assessment frees up capacity within the pre-operative team thereby enabling the assessment of greater numbers of patients with more complex medical and social care needs.

Clearly, telephone pre-assessment has various benefits to patients and healthcare organisations but also has shortfalls. It is difficult to make a thorough patient assessment on the telephone as the ability to notice any non-verbal signals or behaviour is impaired and also baseline observations cannot be checked and recorded. Besides, some patients may be unfamiliar or uncomfortable with telephone assessment, which could make them nervous or provoke uncharacteristic responses.

It is therefore important to notify patients prior to telephone assessment and also solicit their consent. Care should be taken to verify the correct patient is contacted and also to ensure confidentiality. Healthcare professionals involved in telephone pre-assessment need to be well trained and should utilise structured written questionnaires necessary to determine patient suitability for day surgery and anaesthetic. Questionnaires should be kept short and simple to maintain patients' interest and cooperation.

Provision of adequate information is also necessary to enable patients to make appropriate arrangements for admission, discharge and post-operative care at home. Thorough patient education via the phone is essential to facilitate patients' readiness for surgery, good understanding of the procedure, what to expect on the day of surgery as well as discharge and after care.

One-stop cataract surgery

One-stop cataract surgery

The ever-increasing demand for cataract surgery calls for measures to reduce waiting times for patients to undergo surgery. Traditionally, the majority of patients with cataract in England are seen by their optometrist and referred to their primary physician who then refers them to the hospital for an ophthalmologist assessment and consideration for surgery. There is however considerable variation in waiting times amongst NHS organisations, with a median waiting time of 70 days (Wood, 2007). The waiting time for a patient to have cataract surgery varies from consultant to consultant within the same NHS trust and also varies from trust to trust due to the different demands (e.g. case loads and time schedules for patients to be booked into consultant clinics and for pre-operative assessment by nurses) along the patient pathway. The rate of cataract day-cases is also as high as 100 per cent in some units and as low as 74 per cent in others (NHS Institute for Innovation and Improvement, 2008). Clearly the need for one-stop cataract surgery cannot be over-emphasised, as NHS organisations in England are also required to see and treat patients within 18 weeks from the time of referral (NHS Improvement Plan, 2004).

NHS Executive (2000) describes one-stop cataract surgery as an innovative scheme where the optometrist or primary physician makes the diagnosis of a cataract and books the patient direct on to a theatre list, thereby bypassing all the stages and processes which vary from NHS trust to trust. One-stop cataract surgery clearly reduces unnecessary waits by shortening the referral to treatment time as well as reducing variations amongst NHS in terms of different demands along the pathway. NHS Institute for Innovation and Improvement (2008) argues that direct referral from optometrist or primary physician to hospital eye services has the following advantages:

Patient-centred benefits:

- Reduces hospital attendance from three visits to one and also offers patients their date for surgery right from the outset. Reducing hospital attendance from three to one is particularly beneficial to the elderly who may have poor mobility and vision and thus be dependent on others for transport.
- Shorter waiting time for surgery as non-value-added steps are removed from the referral process.

Organisational benefits:

- Reduces administrative workload of primary physicians as well as workload associated with waiting list procedures.
- Correct referrals saves unnecessary clinic visit by patients thereby freeing up space for other patients to be seen.

Despite the various benefits of one-stop cataract surgery, it has shortfalls. The issue of 'false positive referrals' leads to cancellation of surgery and waste of theatre time. The unpredictable problems associated with unscreened patients with a previous history of trauma or dense cataract can also be counterproductive in terms of anticipated patient and organisational benefits (Hughes *et al.*, 2001; Vallance and Dhillon, 2005). There is also the issue of consent. It has been suggested that one-stop cataract surgery pressurises patients to go ahead with surgery as it may not offer them enough time or 'cooling off' period to enable them to make informed decisions regarding the proposed surgery (Hughes *et al.*, 2001; Gaskell *et al.*, 2001). The success of one-stop cataract surgery will depend on the diagnostic skills of referring optometrists and primary physicians to reduce 'false positive referrals' as well as experienced surgeons and anaesthetists to deal with problems associated with unscreened patients. In view of the short-falls associated with one-stop cataract surgery some evidence suggests a two-stop model where one visit will be for diagnosis and pre-operative assessment, and a second visit for surgery (NHS Executive, 2000; Vallance and Dhillon, 2005; NHS Institute for Innovation and Improvement, 2008).

Conclusion

The provision of quality day-case surgery requires attention to detail at every step of the patient pathway, including pre-operative assessment. Effective pre-operative assessment identifies essential resources for successful day-case cataract surgery, improves planned admission processes and also contributes to efficiency and productivity of the organisation, as well as enhancing patient experience and the clinical process. However, healthcare professionals should utilise evidence-based protocols to deliver patient care. Clearly, efficient and effective provision of day-case cataract surgery requires that pre-operative assessment is considered alongside a good patient referral and booking system, successful day surgical outcome and appropriate post-operative care at home. It is important to give patients emergency telephone numbers to enable them to contact the hospital in case of any queries, clarifications, or treatment of any complication associated with the surgery. Prompt and appropriate management of post-operative complications is vital to restore vision. The management of post-operative complications via the ophthalmic accident and emergency department is explored in more detail in Chapter 3.

References

Allan, B. (2001). 'Cataract surgery: Patient preparation and surgical technique.' *Optometry Today* (July Issue): 28–33.

Assia, E., Raskin, T., Kaiserman, I., Rotenstreich, Y., and Segev, F. (1998). 'Effect of aspirin intake on bleeding during cataract surgery.' *Journal of Cataract and Refractive Surgery* 24 (9): 1243–6.

Association of Anaesthetists of Great Britain and Ireland (2005). *Day Surgery*. London: AAGBI.

British National Formulary (2007). *Number 54 (Aspirin)*. London: BMJ and RPS Publishing Group.

Chang, D., and Campbell, J. (2005). 'Intraoperative floppy iris syndrome associated with tamsulosin.' *Journal of Cataract and Refractive Surgery* 31: 664–73.

Dewsbury, C. (2003). *Warfarin: Drug Interactions*. London: Royal Pharmaceutical Society of Great Britain.

Dick, M. (2005). *Patient Group Directions Policy*. South Tees Hospital NHS Trust.

Digner, M. (2007). 'At your convenience: Preoperative assessment by telephone.' *Journal of Perioperative Practice* 17 (7): 294–300.

Funnell, M., and Anderson, R. (2004). 'Empowerment and self-management of diabetes.' *American Diabetes Association* 22 (3): 123–7.

Gaskell, A., McLaughlin, A., Young, E., and McCristal, K. (2001). 'Direct referral of cataract patients into a pilot one-stop cataract surgery facility.' *Journal of Royal College of Surgery, Edinburgh*, 46: 133–7.

Healthcare Commission (2005). *Acute Hospital Portfolio Review: Day Surgery*. London: Commission for Healthcare Audit and Inspection.

Heath, H. (2000). 'The nurse's role in assessing older people.' *Elderly Care* 12 (1): 23–4.

Hirschman, D., and Morby, L. (2006). 'A study of the safety of continued anticoagulation for cataract surgery patients.' *Nursing Forum* 41 (1): 30–7.

Hughes, E.H., Forrest, F., and Diamond, J.P. (2001). '"One-stop" cataract surgery: The Bristol Eye Hospital experience 1997–1999.' *Eye* 15: 306–8.

Konstantos, A. (2001). 'Anticoagulation and cataract surgery: A review of the literature.' *Anaesthetic Intensive Care* 29: 11–18.

Medicines and Health Regulatory Agency (2006). 'Current problems in pharmacovigilence.' *Drug Safety: Bulletin* 31: 6–7.

Mitchell, M. (1999). 'Patient's perception of day surgery: A literature review.' *Ambulatory Surgery* 8 (1): 19–29.

Mitchell, M. (2002). 'Guidance for the psychological care of day case surgery patients.' *Nursing Standard* 16 (40): 41–3.

NHS Executive (2000). *Action on Cataracts: Good Practice Guidance.* London: DoH.

NHS Improvement Plan (2004). *Putting People at the Heart of Public Services.* London: DoH.

NHS Institute for Innovation and Improvement (2008). *Focus on: Cataracts (Delivery Quality and Value).* London: DoH.

NHS Modernisation Agency (2002a). *National Good Practice Guidance on Pre-operative Assessment for Day Surgery: Operating Theatre & Pre-operative Assessment Programme.* London: DoH.

NHS Modernisation Agency (2002b). *Step Guide to Improving Operating Theatre Performance: NHS Modernisation Agency Theatre Programme.* London: DoH.

NHS Modernisation Agency (2004). *Day Surgery: A Good Practice Guide.* London: DoH.

NMC (2002). *Guidelines for Administration of Medicines: Patient Group Directions.* London: NMC.

Picton, C., Granby, T., Joshua, A., and Johnson, W. (2004). *Patient Group Directions.* Manchester: National Prescribing Centre.

Orem, D. (1995). *Nursing: Concepts of Practice*, 5th edn. St. Louis: Mosby.

Roper, N., Logan, W. W., and Tierney, A. J. (2000). *The Roper-Logan-Tierney Model of Nursing: Based on Activities of Daily Living.* Edinburgh: Elsevier Health Sciences.

Rotenstreich, Y., Rubowitz, A., Segev, F., Jaesger-Roslu, S., and Assia, E. (2001). 'Effect of warfarin therapy on bleeding during cataract surgery.' *Journal of Cataract and Refractive Surgery* 27 (9): 1344–5.

Royal College of Anaesthetists (2006). *Raising the Standard: A Compendium of Audit Recipes (Pre-admission assessment).* Accessed on 12.09.2007 from: www.rcoa.ac.uk/index.asp?PageID

Royal College of Anaesthetists and Royal College of Ophthalmologists (2001). *Local Anaesthesia for Intraocular Surgery.* Accessed on 12.09.2007 from: www.rcophth.ac.uk/docs/publications/localAnaesthesia.pdf

Royal College of Ophthalmologists (2004). *Cataract Surgery Guidelines.* London: Royal College Ophthalmologists.

Stanford, P. (1998). 'Patients assessment for ophthalmic patients.' *Nursing Standard* 12 (44): 49–55.

Tannahill, A., and Downie, R.S. (1990). *Health Promotion: Models and Values.* Oxford: Oxford Medical Press.

Valance, J.H., and Dhillon, B. (2005). 'Preoperative assessment of cataract surgery patients.' *Journal of Cataract and Refractive Surgery* 31: 1083–4.

Vasavada, A., and Singh, R. (2000). 'Phacoemulsification in eyes with small pupil.' *Journal of Cataract and Refractive Surgery* 26: 1210–18.

Walsgrove, H. (2006). 'Putting education into practice for pre-operative patient assessment.' *Nursing Standard* 20 (47): 35–9.

Wood, C. (2007). 'Surgery for cataract.' *British Medical Journal* 334 (7585): 107.

Chapter 3

Eye emergencies – Accident and Emergency ophthalmic practice

Ramesh Seewoodhary

Ophthalmic triage and decision-making
Purpose of triage
Categories of triage
The triage process
The triage of children
Telephone triage and ethical considerations
Effective decision-making
The red eye – categories and management
Eye injuries and patient care
Patient decision-making and the use of the
Health Belief Model

Introduction

Chapter 2 explored the importance of pre-operative assessment and day-case cataract surgery, and also stressed the significance and relevance of utilising evidence-based protocols as a basis for ophthalmic management and care. The ensuing discussion in this chapter again reinforces this issue, but with particular emphasis on ophthalmic emergencies. Following day-case cataract surgery, some patients may develop severe postoperative complications such as acute iridocyclitis, conjunctivitis, or raised intra-ocular pressure. Such conditions are classified as ocular emergencies and would require immediate ophthalmic treatment to prevent sight loss.

This chapter aims to provide an insight into the current issues and future challenges surrounding ophthalmic emergencies and the care and management of patients in the Accident and Emergency department. Acute ophthalmic problems are also encountered in other care settings such as occupational health centres, and the community, for example, schools, leisure centres, paediatric units, general practice and care of the elderly.

Patients presenting with an ocular emergency are most anxious about sight loss. Ophthalmic trauma accounts for 6% of all emergencies seen in the Accident and Emergency department. Health practitioners must identify those patients who require urgent care as early management may prevent sight loss and help to promote visual recovery.

Clearly, the healthcare practitioner may encounter many challenges and dilemmas in this ophthalmic setting. Within the current National Health Service (NHS) climate any wrong decision or incompetent care will constitute negligence resulting in medico-legal implications. As healthcare practitioners are taking on more roles and responsibilities, awareness of the legal pitfalls in practice is imperative. A sound knowledge and understanding of the application of the law and ethics to professional practice are therefore essential to safeguard the best interests of ophthalmic patients and maintain professional standards. Indeed, the legal and ethical issues related to professional practice are discussed at length and with application to ophthalmic practice in Chapter 8 of this book.

The challenges around ophthalmic triage and effective decision-making in a wider context including children will be examined. This chapter will also explore the issues around the management of the different categories of the red eye. The last section examines ocular injuries and patient care. Thinking points have also been included within this chapter to stimulate learning and thinking.

Ophthalmic triage and decision-making

Ophthalmic triage

In the Accident and Emergency department, the ophthalmic practitioner must be able to differentiate between patients whose needs are urgent and those who do not need immediate attention. Marsden (1999) defines this system of prioritising as triage. This involves clinical judgements that have to be made within a short span of time (Cioffi, 1999). The conditions which affect patients attending with sight problems are very varied (York and Proud, 1990).

Initial assessment, if taken as a process to screen out patients with immediately life-threatening conditions, is triage in its purest form (Buchan et al., 2003). All triage assessment should be based on a holistic approach, taking into account the patient's psychological and physiological well-being (Crouch, 1994). This initial process involves:

a. Visualisation of the patient, assessing the airway, breathing, circulation followed by a brief head-to-toe scan of the patient observing for physical signs of illness or injury.

b. Exploration and identification of the presenting complaint. Asking the patient what, how and when.

c. Triage decision – direct patient to clinical area to receive care or to registration. Brief documentation of presenting complaint and triage decision are very important.

Jones (1988) further elaborates that triage is the immediate or early assessment and prioritisation, by trained personnel, of the need for patients to be examined by a doctor, to prevent harmful delays. Failure to identify an ophthalmic emergency may endanger patients' sight, particularly in cases of vascular problems which may deteriorate quickly and whose symptoms are not obvious to non-medical personnel. An example is a patient attending with a central retinal artery occlusion, which is painless and vision may be severely reduced to hand movements. Effective triaging and early emergency intervention may help restore vision if the patient attends immediately within 30–60 minutes. York and Proud (1990) clearly point out that failure to identify urgency can lead to a patient suffering from a potentially blinding condition finding himself at the wrong end of a long queue in the Accident and Emergency department. With high attendance rates and over 70% of patients attending being non-urgent, the nurse must ensure that patients are triaged within five minutes of their arrival (DoH 1995). The 1995 Patient's Charter has been influential on nurse triage; its fifth standard states that 'you will be seen immediately and your need for treatment assessed'. Crouch (1994) states that the NHS Management Executive has defined 'immediate' to mean within five minutes of arrival. Thus triage is seen as an integral part of providing a quality service and is recognised as a way of establishing immediate contact between patient and nurse, initiating care and improving communication.

The purpose of triage

The purpose of triage

Triage is required to categorise ophthalmic patients correctly and provide appropriate care at the correct time in order to prevent permanent loss of vision. Triage, initially developed by military surgeons to deal with the large number of war casualties, is designed to ensure that patients with conditions requiring urgent treatment are seen first. Banerjee *et al.* (1998) conclude that a system of patient categorisation must be in place when attending to patients with ophthalmic conditions. The success of patient prioritisation depends, however, on adequate training of nurses and clear guidelines for each category being readily available. It is important that the triage system is explained to all casualty attendees to prevent the perception that some patients are 'jumping the queue'.

Categories of triage

Categories of triage

Essentially, there are three categories of triage. These are:

1) emergency

2) urgent

3) non-urgent.

The emergency category warrants immediate initiation and evaluation of medical and nursing care prior to registration. Every minute of delay can result in irreversible visual loss. This category includes sudden painless loss of vision caused by a central retinal artery occlusion and severe chemical burns which can be alkaline or acidic. Early nursing and medical intervention can make a great difference in the patient's visual outcome.

Urgent category patients need to be seen by a doctor as soon as possible but a slight delay of a few minutes should not make the condition worse. These include penetrating eye injuries, primary closed angle glaucoma, retinal detachment, acute anterior uveitis, corneal abrasions, corneal foreign bodies, arc eye, hyphaema, blunt trauma, corneal ulceration and scleritis.

The non-urgent category which is the largest group of patients account for over 70% of patients who attend a dedicated ophthalmic Accident and Emergency department (York and Proud, 1990). Their presence could mask the very small number of patients for whom urgent emergency treatment is essential. Such categories include minor eye irritations, cystic conditions and long standing vague symptoms. The latter includes history of gradually diminishing vision e.g. cataracts.

The triage process

The triage process

The ophthalmic triage process need not be a time consuming task in a busy acute healthcare setting. Knowledge and experience are two main prerequisites in ensuring patients' safety on arrival or until they leave the department. The system effectively works as follows.

When the patient arrives in the Accident and Emergency department or presents at any acute healthcare setting, the triage nurse obtains a verbal history from the patient. Buchan *et al.* (2003) advocate that nurses trained in slit-lamp examination can provide an effective service for the safe diagnosis and treatment of common eye problems. Box 3.1 outlines the practical and useful questions to ask.

Box 3.1

Taking a history from a patient with an ocular problem

Five baseline questions are asked:

1. What is your present eye complaint?
2. When did it start?
3. Is your vision affected?
4. Do you have any medical problem and known allergies?
5. Are you presently taking any medication?

Continued overleaf

If there is a history of trauma, then the following must be asked and noted:

a. What were you doing at the time before the accident?

b. How did it happen?

c. Were you using any power tool?

d. Were you wearing goggles/safety glasses?

e. What first aid treatment did you receive?

In the case of chemical injuries, the following must be asked and noted:

a. What chemical was splashed into your eye(s)?

b. How did this happen?

c. When did this happen?

d. What first aid treatment was carried out?

e. Has the injury affected your sight ?

For patients presenting with contact lens related eye problems, a thorough history will aid in problem identification and treatment. Some of the questions asked will include:

a. What type of lenses are you wearing?

b. Do you have redness, pain, itching or discharge?

c. Is your vision blurred?

d. Are you unusually sensitive to bright light?

e. When did you first notice the problem?

f. Did you go to another physician or try to treat it yourself?

g. What solutions do you use?

h. Did you fall asleep with your lenses in?

i. Were you handling chemicals or hot peppers?

j. Do the lenses film up quickly or slip under your lids when you blink?

The triage of children

The triaging policy must also consider the special needs of children for priority (Bentley, 1995). The RCN considers the triage nurse to be influential in the care of the child and family because this nurse will be their first point of contact. A child's condition can worsen quickly and the strangeness of the A&E environment may exacerbate children's fears and anxieties.

The triage of children in A&E is a challenging duty and the triage nurse must be legally supported by a qualified paediatric nurse for medico-legal reasons. All children presenting with an eye problem must be seen by a doctor. The role of the nurse in supporting the child and family is important throughout the child's journey in the A&E Department.

Eye injuries are a leading cause of visual impairment and monocular blindness in children. Kutschke (1994) finds possible causes of eye injuries in children to be ubiquitous. They commonly occur at home, at school and in play areas. Early identification and treatment are both essential as York and Proud (1990) point out that children and their families should be given priority.

Orbital cellulitis is a severe infection of the orbital tissues which may involve the eye and can cause brain abscesses if treatment is delayed. A child presenting with such a systemic disorder will be unwell, pyrexial and lethargic. Long waiting in the A&E Department is not advisable as orbital cellulitis can cause the child's condition to worsen by the minute. Phillips and Robson (1992) emphasise the necessity for prompt triage of children, who are frequently brought into the department by their parents. It can easily be assumed that such patients require less than urgent attention simply because they have not arrived by ambulance. Action for Sick Children reinforces Department of Health guidelines which recommend that there are 'effective procedures to prioritise waiting children and ensure that they are seen promptly' (DoH, 1991). A newborn baby up to 21 days old who presents with purulent conjunctivitis requires prompt treatment as some pathogens are known to cause corneal perforation within 36 hours, e.g. *Neisseria gonorrhoeae*.

It is recommended by Alcock *et al.* (1985) that children who attend with non-emergency disorders be given access to a staff member who can provide play and information about the impending treatment. This is applicable to children who attend the A&E with styes, chalazion, blepharitis or an allergic eye disorder.

Telephone triage and ethical considerations

Telephone triage

Effective telephone triage is a vital component of problem diagnosis in the ambulatory care setting. Stetson (1986) stresses the primary goal of telephone triage is to assist the patient in obtaining an effective and timely resolution to his or her problem. The first encounter with a patient is likely to be over the phone. In such an instance the nurse does not have the advantage of being able to observe the patient and make an assessment about his or her condition. It is up to the nurse to elicit meaningful information from the patient and formulate a working diagnosis based on the patient's symptoms.

When a patient calls with an ophthalmic problem, it is important to note that it is a problem to him or her and it does not matter whether the nurse has already talked to many patients that morning with the same symptoms. From the patient perspective his or her problem is unique. Stetson (1986) offers useful guidelines to telephone triage.

The following points are helpful:

1. Remember it is a problem unique to the patient.

2. Listen for the symptoms.

3. Listen to what the patient is saying.

4. Ascertain the chief complaint; explore nature of the symptoms.

5. Obtain the best possible history – note: duration, onset, vision.

6. Stay calm and reassure patient.

Note down all information for medico-legal reasons (Seewoodhary, 2003). The ultimate goal is to assist the patient to obtain an effective and timely resolution to his or her problem. With good information the nurse will be better able to advise the patient. Obtaining a clear, concise history will assist in establishing a preliminary diagnosis. The practitioner will need to work within a given protocol and keep accurate records and at the same time the practitioner must exercise his or her professional judgement.

Ophthalmic triaging is a great responsibility in any acute care setting. Triage involves the use of high-level assessment skills and Parmar and Hewitt (1985) suggest that a trained nurse ought to be the named triage nurse. McDonald *et al.* (1995) highlight that triage has ethical implications and is part of the duty of care which a healthcare professional owes to his or her patient.

Evidence-based care integrated within the triage system has many benefits. It makes the patients feel safe and well cared for in an anxiety-provoking environment. Every second counts when triaging patients with real eye emergency conditions. Failure and delay in identifying and treating an ophthalmic emergency can progress to irreparable sight loss.

Effective decision-making

Effective decision-making

Effective triaging requires effective decision-making, Thompson *et al.* (2004) identify that mistakes in the planning and execution of clinical decisions are a major factor in adverse events occurring in the NHS. Seven to ten per cent of patients suffer some form of adverse event and most are considered preventable.

Improving decision-making is one strategy to prevent errors when triaging, especially when working under conditions of irreducible uncertainty. Thompson *et al.* (2004) argued that irreducible uncertainty means having to make decisions in less than ideal circumstances. Triaging allows the ophthalmic practitioner to have early patient contact in the Accident and Emergency department. The impact of the ophthalmic nurse's role should never be underestimated, as prioritising patients is essential to prevent sight loss. Prioritising accurately by taking a pertinent history and carrying out an eye examination will ensure that the patient is correctly managed in the department.

THINKING POINT

TAKE A FEW MINUTES TO REFLECT ON THE FOLLOWING:

a. What are the possible clinical uncertainties the nurse might encounter when carrying out prioritisation of patients who attend with an ophthalmic problem in an Accident and Emergency department?

a. What are the challenges of decision-making when triaging ophthalmic patients in a busy general Accident and Emergency department?

a. What ethical dilemmas might occur when carrying out telephone triage for an ophthalmic patient ?

The red eye – categories and management

Eye disease is estimated to account for between 40 and 50 general practice consultations per 1000. According to Falcon (1989) about 30% of these patients are diagnosed as having infectious conjunctivitis and another 30% as having allergic conjunctivitis. An acute red eye, in the absence of specialist facilities, can prove difficult to identify and manage. Duguid (1997) stresses that accurate diagnosis is essential in order to initiate appropriate treatment, especially as there are many possible causes of red eye. Red eye associated with pain and photophobia can be sight threatening if it is misdiagnosed or wrongly treated.

The 'red eye' can range from a mild ophthalmic disorder where vision is unimpaired to a severely painful condition with severe visual loss at initial presentation. Davey (1996) points out some symptoms are helpful as they point the way to a diagnosis, while others need clarification to understand precisely what the patient means.

Blurred vision

This may result from a reduction of visual acuity, or diplopia, or simply a need for a change in glasses. Mucus strands can smear across the vision and clear on blinking. The latter can be caused by bacterial conjunctivitis, allergic conjunctivitis, dry eyes or even chronic lid inflammatory disorder such as blepharitis.

Haloes

These may refer to the glare or dazzle seen in cataracts. Coloured or rainbow haloes suggest corneal oedema which is present in primary acute closed angle glaucoma, so if it is associated with pain the patient requires urgent referral to an ophthalmologist. Patients referring to ghosting of images instead of haloes may need to see their optometrist for refraction.

Photophobia

This is dislike of bright light which can be caused by an acute inflammatory eye disorder such as acute iritis, or acutely raised intra-ocular pressure as in primary acute closed angle glaucoma.

Corneal abrasions or ulceration are also accompanied by redness and intense photophobia. Photophobia without a red eye is usually seen in migraine and raised intracranial pressure.

Pain

Pain as opposed to discomfort and soreness suggest a serious cause. Pain around the red eye and at the back of the eye may suggest an acute iritis or severe scleritis. Pain that radiates around the red eye and forehead and associated with nausea and vomiting usually indicates an abnormally raised intra-ocular pressure such as a primary acute angle closure glaucoma. Severe pain on the scalp and forehead accompanied by a rash may indicate herpes zoster ophthalmicus. The pain usually comes first and this is followed by a rash a few days later. The patient's eye may be red and sticky but if accompanied by photophobia he or she must be referred to an ophthalmologist urgently.

Grittiness

A patient who complains of grittiness and mild bilateral red eyes may be suffering from chronic dry eyes and occasionally blepharitis.

Foreign body sensation

This is a common symptom among many patients who present with a red eye. The cause can be an actual foreign body or corneal abrasion or an in-growing eyelash or dry eyes.

Sticky discharge

Purulent yellow or greenish sticky discharge occurs as a result of bacterial infection such as conjunctivitis or occasionally blepharitis. Mucousy discharge may be a classical feature of seasonal conjunctivitis or an acute allergic reaction.

Itchy eyes

Constant itchiness may be due to allergy, conjunctivitis, dry eyes and blepharitis. Patients with skin disorders such as eczema are more likely to rub their eyelids constantly in order to alleviate the itchiness. Consequently chronic red eye is a common association in patients with atopic disorder.

Judge (1992) states that taking a thorough history is the most important step in evaluating a red eye. The key questions to ask are:

a. How long has the eye been red?

b. Is the eye painful or sore?

c. Is there a yellow purulent discharge?

d. Does the eye water?

e. Is there any light sensitivity (photophobia)?

f. Does the eye itch?

g. Is there a past history of eye problems or a red eye?

h. Is the vision blurred?

i. Has there been a recent injury or foreign body?

j. Are any family members affected?

k. Has the patient instilled any drops or ointment which has made the eye red, itchy, puffy or watery?

It is important briefly to enquire into the patient's medical history, drug history and social history as these are also highly relevant in identifying the cause of the red eye. A logical and systematic method of examination will assist differential diagnosis. The procedure outlined below provides a checklist and sound framework for identification of red eye. The salient clinical features and causes of red eyes will be described and illustrated in the context of the condition in which they occur. The equipment required is listed in Table 3.1.

Table 3.1

Examination equipment and drops

Equipment	Snellen's chart
	Pinhole occluder
	Torch (with blue light filter)
	Fluorescein strips
	Ophthalmoscope
	Cotton bud
Drops	Benoxinate (local anaesthetic)
	Tropicamide 1% (to dilate the pupils)
	Saline 0.9% (to moisten fluorescein strip)

Visual acuity is assessed and tested separately for distance vision using a Snellen's chart. Corrected distance glasses must be worn. Normal vision is 6/6, but if visual acuity is 6/9 or less, vision must be tested using a pinhole occluder. If vision improves with a pinhole occluder, this may suggest a refractive error (Davey, 1996).

If the eye is red and painful and has reduced visual acuity, a serious cause should be sought. Visual acuity measurement must be done accurately as this has medico-legal implications (Seewoodhary, 1983).

A pen torch with strong illumination is helpful to identify most common external eye problems, but slit lamp biomicroscopy provides more detailed examination with good accuracy of diagnosis.

Examine ocular structures in sequence, anterior to posterior, paying particular attention to the following clinical features:

a. Eyelids and lashes – look for lid swelling (stye, chalazion, abscess, allergy) in-growing eyelashes, red eyelid rims with crustiness (blepharitis), redness of the eye and pattern of redness and presence of pus (bacterial infection).

b. Conjunctiva – pattern of redness of the conjunctiva, episclera and sclera may indicate a subconjunctival haemorrhage, or inflammatory disorders such as episcleritis and scleritis.

c. Cornea – shine torch on the cornea and observe brightness of light reflection. If the reflection is cloudy or hazy in the presence of a painful red eye, look for serious cause such as corneal ulcer or primary acute angle closure glaucoma. Staining with fluorescein may show a corneal abrasion if a cobalt blue filter is used.

d. Anterior Chamber – examine for depth, hypopyon, hyphaema or a flat anterior chamber. A slit lamp beam will show cells and flare which are inflammatory products seen in acute iritis.

e. Iris – observe for contours, colour, new vessels formation, dialysis and lesions. In iritis the colour of the iris is muddy and blood vessels are engorged and easily visible with a slit lamp.

f. Pupil – observe for pupil size, shape, outline, and reaction to light. In primary acute angle closure glaucoma, the pupil is mid-dilated and does not react to light at all. In iritis the pupil size is smaller due to spasm of the sphincter pupillary muscles and swelling of the iris. The pupillary reaction is present but it is sluggish. Adhesion of the iris to the lens is commonly seen in acute iritis and this gives the pupil a scallop appearance.

f. Redness – note if the red eye is unilateral or bilateral.
Redness all over the conjunctiva associated with severe pain and photophobia may indicate either an acute glaucoma or an acute iritis.
Redness associated with mild pain or discomfort may indicate conjunctivitis, episcleritis, dry eye or an allergy.
Redness around the corneal limbus indicates either a corneal disease, uveitis, or raised intra-ocular pressure.
Intense velvety redness with severe ocular pain is commonly a feature of severe anterior scleritis.

The eyes should be palpated through closed lids to assess intraocular pressure

A normal eye can be slightly indented between forefingers through the upper lid while the patient is instructed to look down. In acute glaucoma the affected eye feels stony hard. The normal eye must be palpated first for comparison. Finally, palpate the pre-auricular nodes beside the ears. Swollen and tender pre-auricular nodes may be indicative of a viral conjunctivitis or chlamydial conjunctivitis.

Specific ocular conditions

Specific conditions

In this section only common specific 'red eye' conditions will be presented.

Subconjunctival haemorrhage

Subconjunctival haemorrhage is characterised by the striking appearance of a usually flat, red haemorrhage beneath the conjunctiva. Duguid (1997) identifies this condition as extremely common and occurs due to spontaneous rupture of a conjunctival or episcleral capillary as illustrated in Figure 3.1.

It is often precipitated by coughing or physical straining. It may also follow trauma and if, for example, the patient has been using a hammer and chisel or power tools this may be indicative of a perforating injury and intraocular foreign body (Seewoodhary, 2003). In case of head injury, blood from a fracture at the base of the skull may travel through the floor of the orbit to the subconjunctival space.

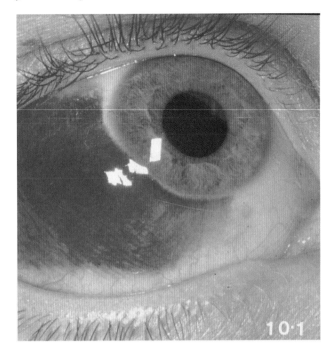

Figure 3.1

Spontaneous subconjunctival haemorrhage
With kind permission of Moorfields Eye Hospital Medical Photography Department
Taken from Seewoodhary, R. (2003) *Ophthalmic Nursing*

Spontaneous subconjunctival haemorrhage is asymptomatic. The patient may first become aware of the condition when informed by an associate, or looking into a mirror. Traumatic subconjunctival haemorrhage may be associated with damage in other parts of the eye which may result in visual disturbance. Coughing and constipation may cause a rise in intra-thoracic pressure resulting in bleeding. Wilson (1986) found that the disorder can also be caused by febrile illnesses and infection such as pneumococcal infection, adenoviruses and epidemic haemorrhagic keratoconjunctivitis. The pattern of redness may be localised or diffused but, in head trauma, the haemorrhage does not have a definable margin posteriorly, but extends backwards into the orbit.

When a bilateral subconjunctival haemorrhage is present, care must be taken to rule out blood dyscrasia (Pau,1978). Spontaneous subconjunctival haemorrhage usually occurs unilaterally, while that following fracture of the skull involves both eyes.

61

No specific treatment is required and the patient will need reassurance that the haemorrhage will disperse over 2 to 3 weeks and may recur without warning. Hypertension and diabetes mellitus should be excluded or investigated. Drops are not indicated and in the absence of trauma referral is not required. Suspected perforating eye injuries should not be palpated as this may cause further intra-ocular complications, e.g. vitreous loss, detached retina or the risk of introducing infection into the eye contents. All patients, therefore, who present with a subconjunctival haemorrhage need careful and thorough evaluation.

Conjunctivitis

Conjunctivitis is a common and usually benign cause of red eyes. Acute conjunctivitis is characterised by a discharge or eyelid stickiness which is often worse on waking up. It causes a red eye from conjunctival injection and foreign body sensation of less than a few weeks duration (Judge, 1992). It is commonly bilateral and bacterial in origin. Unilateral conjunctivitis is more common in children and may be caused by *Streptococcus pneumoniae, Haemophilus influenzae* and *Staphylococcus aureus*. Bilateral purulent red eyes in the newborn require urgent referral and treatment as the cause may be *Neisseria gonorrhoeae*, or Chlamydia. Figure 3.2 shows the seriousness of gonococcal conjunctivitis and a delay in starting treatment may lead to corneal rupture (Jatla and Zhao, 2008).

A blocked tear duct in infants will cause a red eye. If pressure is applied over the naso-lacrimal sac, pus will be expressed from the lacrimal puncta at the medial ends of the eyelids. A purulent dacryocystitis is usually evident in children with blocked tear ducts. Many causes are mild and respond well to broad spectrum antibiotics. The drop of choice is chloramphenicol with fusidic acid 1% a good alternative.

Viral conjunctivitis can affect both adults and children, usually starting in one eye first and becoming bilateral in most cases a few days later. The eyes are red and watery over one to two days. There is history of a recent upper respiratory tract infection. It can also be caused by exposure to a family member or work colleague with red eyes. Epidemic keratoconjunctivitis is a severe viral infection caused by adenovirus types 8 and 19. Unlike other adenoviruses,

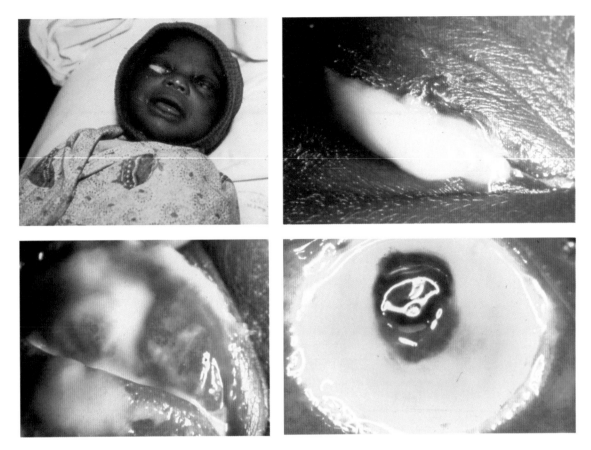

Figure 3.2   **Gonococcal conjunctivitis**
With kind permission of Moorfields Eye Hospital Medical Photography Department

it is not associated with systemic symptoms. The infection may resolve or it may go on to become subepithelial and even stromal and in some cases it becomes chronic (Murray, 1988). The infectious period is two weeks and patients should not go to school or to work during that time. Meticulous hand washing is very important to avoid cross-infection and all work surfaces must be cleaned with alcohol. Swimming in a public pool is prohibited as this has been known to infect other swimmers. A palpable pre-auricular lymph node is strongly supportive of the diagnosis but is present only in about one-fifth of cases (Duguid, 1997).

There is no specific antiviral therapy. A broad spectrum antibiotic is usually prescribed as prophylaxis against a secondary bacterial infection. As the disease is highly contagious, effective health education is essential to avoid infecting others. Towels and face flannels should not be shared and close contact with others should be avoided. Reassurance can be given that the infection may get worse initially before it improves over the following two to three weeks.

Allergic conjunctivitis presents with itching eyes and the onset is bilateral and simultaneous. Unilateral cases may be associated with the use of a particular eye drop. A history of atopy, often asthma or hay fever, and/or a seasonal pattern to recurrences may be obtained.

Vernal conjunctivitis is synonymous with seasonal conjunctivitis associated with intense ocular itching, lacrimation, burning and a stringy discharge noted during spring and summer. Large conjunctivital papillae under the upper lid are seen. Acute exacerbations require topical steroid therapy and this necessitates referral to an ophthalmologist. Mast cell stabilisers such as sodium cromoglycate are useful in preventing future occurrences and not in the acute phase. Susceptible individuals must use the drop prophylactically as the hay season approaches.

Iritis

Iritis is an acute inflammation of the iris. It is often unilateral and the patient complains of a dull, ocular ache. The condition can also exist in a chronic form, often associated with intra-ocular complications such as cataract or glaucoma or both. Photophobia is common and pain on focusing on a near object is less frequently present. Iritis is often associated with rheumatoid diseases or a systemic infection such as tuberculosis. In young adults the cause can be ankylosing spondylitis although in the majority of cases the cause remains unknown.

Vision is often only slightly reduced but if cells and flare are copious in the aqueous humour then vision is reduced markedly. Iritis is characterised by the presence of keratic precipitates which are deposits of cells on the posterior cornea. The pupil is small and may be irregular in outline due to adhesion of the iris to the lens. The pupillary reaction to light is sluggish. The intra-ocular pressure may be below normal, but in some patients it can be elevated. Elevated intra-ocular pressure indicates the onset of secondary glaucoma possibly caused by clogging of the canal of Schlemm by inflammatory debris or by adhesion of the root of the iris to the surface of the cornea. This will result in impairment of aqueous drainage and an iris bombé.

Early treatment is essential to help clear the inflammation to break down any adhesions that are formed between the iris and the lens and to alleviate pain. This should help in the healing process. Cyclopentolate helps to dilate the pupil and this gives symptomatic relief. Topic steroid is also prescribed but with care, since herpetic ulcers can give rise to similar symptoms and occur in anyone. If adhesion is formed between the iris and the lens surface a subconjunctival injection of Mydricaine will be prescribed only if cycloplegic drops fail to break the adhesion. The patient needs to be reviewed regularly to monitor progress in an eye clinic. The wearing of dark glasses offers comfort against bright light. The condition can recur and the patient needs health education as to what course of action to take.

Primary acute angle closure glaucoma:

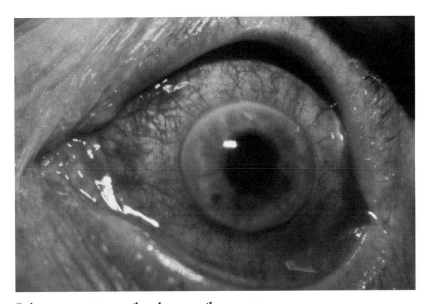

Figure 3.3

Primary acute angle closure glaucoma
With kind permission of Moorfields Eye Hospital Medical Photography Department

Primary acute angle closure glaucoma is usually unilateral, commonly affecting elderly people and is more common in hypermetropes. The corneal diameter tends to be smaller than normal, the iris is anteriorly placed and as the lens swells this pushes the iris forward with a tendency to cause further narrowing of the filtration angle. The onset of an acute attack can be sudden and the disorder is severe. The patient complains of severe unilateral ocular pain associated with headache, nausea, vomiting and blurred vision. The vomiting associated with acute glaucoma may lead to the false diagnosis of acute abdomen. Duguid (1997) states that recent episodes of a milder ocular ache with or without the perception of haloes around lights may be obtained on direct questioning. Haloes are due to corneal oedema as the corneal endothelial pumps fail to function correctly as a result of elevated intra-ocular pressure. These attacks usually occur in the evening or in dim lighting conditions, when the pupil dilates and occludes the drainage angle.

On examination the patient usually looks distressed, nauseated and is reluctant to move. The eye is generally red with marked circumcorneal injection and the cornea looks cloudy in comparison with the fellow eye. The pupil is non-reactive, mid-dilated and oval shaped. The depth of the anterior chamber is very shallow with the root of the iris occluding the drainage filtration angle. The eye becomes severely photophobic and waters a lot. The diagnostic feature is that the eye is hard to palpation in striking contrast to the other eye. Urgent referral to an ophthalmic unit is required and the patient must be given priority as severely raised intra-ocular pressure can cause irreparable visual loss if not treated quickly.

Intravenous acetazolamide 500mg is administered with care, ensuring that the patient is not allergic to sulphonamides. This helps to reduce aqueous outflow by 50–60%. Pilocarpine 2% drops and timolol 0.25% are given ten to twenty minutes following intravenous Diamox. Pilocarpine is an effective miotic which will help draw the congested iris away from the filtration angle, thus increasing aqueous outflow. Timolol is a beta blocker which reduces the rate of aqueous production. All drops must be administered with caution especially as beta blockers are contra-indicated in chronic obstructive airways disease or congestive cardiac failure. The effects of all medications must be monitored and intra-ocular pressure rechecked. The normal baseline intra-ocular pressure is between 12 and 21mm Hg and in an acute attack of glaucoma the intra-ocular pressure can reach 70mm Hg. Once the intra-ocular pressure is brought under control the patient may undergo laser iridotomy, cataract surgery or a peripheral iridectomy as a day-case patient. The sooner the intra-ocular pressure is reduced the less the threat to sight.

THINKING POINT

(These questions are best discussed with a small group of colleagues within the same practice area.)

TAKE A FEW MINUTES TO REFLECT ON THE FOLLOWING:

a. List the causes of red eyes that you have encountered in your clinical practice area.

b. Some causes are not mentioned in this sector. Can you list some other possible causes? How would you prioritise their severity? How can they be recognised?

c. Mismanagement of red eye can be serious and sight threatening. How can this be avoided? (If you have kept a reflective diary, it would be helpful to share and discuss the current issues and challenges you and other colleagues have encountered).

Eye injuries and patient care

Eye injuries and patient care

Eye trauma is a leading cause of significant visual impairment (Bickerton, 2000).

Injuries can be blunt and penetrating and may also involve the lids and orbits. MacCumber (1998) states that eye injuries arise as a result of trauma in five major instances: road traffic accidents, industrial accidents, sport and recreational activities, domestic accidents and assault. Careful evaluation is required by the nurse to ensure accurate assessment of the injury and it is important not to miss any problems that could lead to visual loss or a life threatening situation.

More than 100,000 people in the United States suffer each year from eye trauma (Burlew 1991). Of these individuals, many end up with some permanent vision loss. About 500,000 blinding eye injuries occur yearly worldwide according to MacCumber (1998). Around 85 % of patients are male. MacEwen (1989) shows that the workplace accounts for 69.9% of eye injuries in a 12-month study in 1988–9. The greatest number of eye injuries is within the 20–40 year age group (McGrory, 1996). Between 1997 and 2000 214 people in the UK lost the sight in at least one eye through an industrial injury (Health and Safety Executive, 2001).

Risk taking and its consequences are cited as a main cause of ocular injury (Schmidt and Kramer, 1997) but this is usually unintentionally induced by stress, fatigue, impatience or inadequate knowledge. Falling or tripping is a significant causative factor of eye injury in the elderly, often accompanied with facial trauma and limb fractures. DIY activities constitute similar risk to occupational accidents, sawing, painting, plastering, sanding, etc., according to Milligan (2002). Other domestic injuries include gardening, cleaning products, blunt or penetrating trauma from household items, pets claws or fingernails.

Bickerton (2000) points out that determining the patient's history is a very important first step in evaluating the full extent of the ocular injury. The time allowed for taking a comprehensive history is determined by the severity of the ocular trauma. Disorders requiring immediate treatment such as a patient with a chemical splash in the eyes should be ruled out first. In cases other than a chemical injury, the nurse should have ample time to complete an accurate history and eye examination.

The questions listed in Table 3.2 will help to assess and evaluate the extent and severity of ocular trauma.

Table 3.2

History taking from patients attending with an ocular injury

Question to Ask	Significance
What happened to your eye?	Good starting point to establish the seriousness of the problem
Which eye is involved?	Trauma can be unilateral or bilateral. Assault with chemical can be bilateral. Foreign body while grinding/chiselling can be unilateral.
When did the injury happen?	This influences when to administer first aid or treatment, e.g. chemical injury is irrigated without undue delay.

Where did the injury occur?	This is important as the patient may have had first aid treatment at place of work. Or an assault on the street may prompt you to ask if the police have been informed.
Do you wear glasses or contact lenses?	Glasses may break on impact and result in corneal laceration or intra-ocular foreign body. Contact lenses may retain chemicals in chemical splash eye injury.
Is your vision blurred as a result of the eye injury?	Blurring of vision may signify complications such as corneal abrasion, iritis, cataract, vitreous haemorrhage, macular oedema, retinal tears, optic nerve damage. Arising complication(s) depend largely on the nature of the injury.
Have you instilled any eye drops or ointments?	This is usually serious if the eye injury is perforated and can lead to intra-ocular infection/inflammation.
Have you had a recent eye injury?	A recently operated eye can open on impact, e.g. a fist injury.
Did you wear any protection?	This is a legal requirement at the place of work and preventative in DIY situations.

History taking has medico-legal implications and must also include medical history, medication, drug allergy and family history.

The external eye examination provides information about the overall appearance of facial features around the eyes and of external eye structures. If extreme pain, photophobia, or lid spasm are present, the physician may prescribe an anaesthetic eye drop such as amethocaine 1% which will facilitate the examination. Both eyes must be examined in a systematic way (Bickerton, 2000). See Table 3.3 on page 70.

Table 3.3 **Eye examination following eye injury**

Ocular Structures	What to Observe
Eye lids	Bruises Black eye ptosis Oedema Asymmetry Watery eye Torn puncta Lid laceration
Conjunctiva	Conjunctival haemorrhage Conjunctival laceration Conjunctival injection Conjunctival embedded foreign body
Cornea	Is it clear? Is it oedematous and cloudy? Is it abraded? Is there an embedded foreign body or are there multiple foreign bodies? Is it lacerated deeply, superficially or whole thickness?
Anterior Chamber	Is the anterior chamber present or absent? Is there a hyphaema? Is there a foreign body present?
Iris	Is there a torn iris? Is the iris the same colour on each eye? Is the iris quivering? Is the iris pupillary border regular or irregular?
Pupil	Is the pupil equal and reacting to light in each eye? Is the pupil miosed (traumatic miosis)? Is the pupil larger than normal and does it react very slowly (traumatic mydriasis)? Is there a relative afferent pupillary defect?

The next section will focus on the following:

1. Chemical eye injury

2. Minor trauma

3. Serious closed eye injury

4. Open trauma

5. Ocular trauma in children.

Chemical eye injury

A chemical injury to the eye is a true ophthalmic emergency and nurses and other health care workers need to recognise the importance of prompt and effective treatment (Bickerton, 2000). Glenn (1995) identifies that chemical burns are often associated with crime and unfortunately this type of accident is on the increase. The initial treatment administered by a nurse or a relevant care worker has more impact on visual outcome than any subsequent care from the ophthalmologist.

Chemicals are denoted by their pH value (1–14). This defines them as acid (low pH), alkaline (high pH) or neutral (pH 7). Acids and alkaline chemicals can cause severe disfigurement and blindness. Alkaline agents cause more serious damage than acids as they penetrate deeper. This is due to their hydroxyl ions which combine with fatty acids in cell membranes and cause saponification leading to total disruption and death of cells. Rapid deep penetration will eventually involve the intra-ocular structures (Glenn, 1995). The hydroxyl ions will alter the collagen structures in the cornea, thus making them more prone to damage by degrading enzymes. Alkalis can cause ischaemia and coagulation necrosis of the conjunctiva and sclera.

The most severe alkaline chemicals are:

- magnesium hydroxide
- sodium hydroxide
- potassium hydroxide
- calcium hydroxide
- ammonium hydroxide.

Many of the chemicals are in domestic cleaning products such as oven cleaners and chemical detergents as well as in brick dust, cement and plaster. Ammonium hydroxide is formed in the eye when the patient has been exposed to ammonia gas. This reacts with the tears and has devastating effects. Therefore the patient with a chemical eye injury will not necessarily always present having splashed a liquid directly into the eye. They may have been exposed to a gas. The higher the pH the worse the tissue damage with irreversible damage occurring at pH 11.5. Alkaline solutions penetrate rapidly through the ocular tissues and will continue to cause damage long after the injury is sustained.

The clinical course of alkaline burns can be acute or chronic. In the acute stage the eye can become dry, develop raised intra-ocular pressure, corneal oedema, cataract and corneal anaesthesia. In the chronic stage the cornea can develop new vessels, ulceration and scars. The lid and conjunctiva can become scarred and the lashes can turn in to irritate the cornea. Glaucoma can become uncontrollable and eventually the eye can become blind and painful. A perforated eye can become unsightly and shrunken and may have to be removed.

Acid burns are generally less severe than alkaline burns and tend to improve with treatment and time. Acid damage is limited because the acid combines with the protein of the superficial eye tissue to form a barrier which limits further penetration of the acid. Substances with a pH lower than 7.0 are considered acidic. Examples are sulphuric acid found in car battery fluid and hydrochloric acid commonly used in rust cleaning.

Patients who have been exposed to CS gas (O-Chlorobenzylidene Malononitrile) should be kept in a designated eye treatment area and managed by staff wearing protective clothing against its effects. These patients must not be taken through the waiting room as CS gas vapours on the patient's clothing may cause chemical burns to the eyes of others nearby. The preferred treatment is to blow dry air directly on the eye with an electric fan if available. This helps the dissolved gas to vaporise and the irritation should disappear in minutes. Rinsing the eye without having done this can further induce and prolong the severe burning sensation. The corneal epithelium typically remains intact and vision rapidly returns to normal. All patients are discharged home with a short course of broad spectrum antibiotic eye drops (O'Driscoll *et al.*, 1995).

Glenn (1995) stresses that many health workers may be unaware of the full importance of chemical injuries. Delay in identifying the problem and mistreatment can cause the patient a great deal of distress and visual loss. Any chemical injury must be dealt with urgently and eye irrigation commenced immediately. The history of the event and type of chemical can be obtained while irrigating and any further history gained following irrigation. The pH of the eye is recorded using litmus paper.

Local anaesthetic is recommended for ease of the procedure as well as for patient comfort and co-operation. Normal saline is used to irrigate the eye. Any loose pieces of solid chemical, e.g. cement should be removed from the eye using a cotton bud. Irrigation fluid should run directed from the nasal side to the outer canthus with the patient looking up, down, left and right. The lower lid is pulled down and irrigated. The upper lid must be double everted and irrigated as chemicals can evade washout under the lid. Contact lenses, if worn, must also be removed as these will retain chemicals as well as reducing the effectiveness of washouts. In severe cases both eyes are irrigated simultaneously for about 20 minutes for each eye. The pH of the tears should be checked before and also 3–4 minutes after irrigation. The pH is expected to return to neutral (pH7), if not the irrigation must continue (Bickerton, 2000). Glenn (1995) advocates that the pH levels must be monitored for one hour after irrigation and if the pH rises then irrigation is recommenced until a neutral pH is achieved. The patient's visual acuity must be checked and recorded as a base line to assess the effects of treatment as well as for legal reasons in case of claims for compensation.

After the ocular pH has returned to normal a complete ocular examination should be done to evaluate the extent of tissue damage. A complete blanching of the conjunctiva is an extremely poor diagnostic sign with poor clinical outcome.

Most mild to moderate burns resolve in 7–10 days. Patients may be prescribed cycloplegic drops, e.g. homatropine, to dilate the pupil. This reduces pain caused by ciliary muscle spasm and also prevents posterior synechiae. Vitamin C eye drops, in the form of potassium ascorbate, are prescribed in severe chemical burns as it is a co-factor in collagen synthesis and an antioxidant preventing damage by chemically active free radicals released either from chemical reactions or polymorph enzymes. Vitamin C replacement therapy is considered essential for healing and preventing intra-ocular complications such as cataract and uveitis according to Duffy 2008.

Antibiotics and steroid drops are prescribed in most cases. Patients on steroid therapy need to be monitored regularly to rule out complications such as corneal lysis, glaucoma and secondary infection. If the cornea is severely damaged a soft therapeutic bandage contact lens is used to promote epithelial migration and basement membrane regeneration. The doctor may also prescribe eye lubricant and artificial tears to be used as needed for comfort and promoting healing. Local anaesthetic drops are used only with the irrigation procedure and if necessary during eye examination procedure. It is important to note that repeated topical anaesthetic drops cause epithelial toxicity, prevent re-epithelialisation and can cause corneal ulcers and scarring (Hooper, 1997). Davis and Ali (1997) found that prolonged treatment with steroids when used in conjunction with topical vitamin C is not associated with corneoscleral melting.

Treatment intervention and prognosis are both influenced by the degree of limbal ischaemia. The grading system for the severity of chemical burns is provided in Table 3.4.

Table 3.4

Grading systems for severity of chemical burns

From Roper-Hall (1965) and Randleman (2006)

Grade	Corneal Haze	Epithelium	Limba Ischaemia	Prognosis
(i)	Nil	subtotal loss	Nil	Full recovery
(ii)	Mild to moderate	subtotal loss	$< 1/3$	Recovery, minor scarring
(iii)	Iris details obscured	Total loss	$1/3 - 1/2$	Significant visual loss
(iv)	Opaque	Total loss	$> 1/2$	Risk of loss of eye

In the case of an ocular chemical burn, time is of the essence. Immediate irrigation with bland fluids is essential until the pH remains between 7.3 and 7.7. Chemical injuries to the eye can be devastating and mismanagement can result in visual impairment. All healthcare staff must be instructed on correct techniques of eye irrigation. The public must be made aware of the dangers of chemical in the eyes through health education. Sight is precious and an astute health professional can have a huge impact on a patient's vision.

Minor trauma

Minor eye injuries are localised on the ocular surface and can be managed effectively. The outer coats of the eye provide an excellent barrier against trauma and infection, however Forrester *et al.* (1996) state that if the cornea is damaged infection can occur. Minor trauma includes the following:

- Corneal abrasion
- Recurrent corneal abrasion
- Ultra violet light injury
- Conjunctival abrasion and foreign body
- Subtarsal foreign body
- Corneal foreign body.

Corneal abrasion

Corneal abrasion is a very common condition. The epithelial layer is exposed and is easily damaged by the intruding finger of a baby, branch, flying object etc. The eye waters profusely, photophobia is common, and the pain is severe.

Topical anaesthetic is required to ease the pain and for assessment of the patient while in the emergency department. Repeated use of topical anaesthesia is dangerous as it inhibits healing and thus should only be used in the department. The patient's visual acuity must be recorded accurately for medico-legal reasons.

Exposed corneal nerves, when damaged, cause ciliary muscle spasm and pain as there is a close association between the trigeminal sensory nerves of both the cornea and the ciliary body muscles. By dilating the pupil with a cycloplegic agent, e.g. homatropine 2%, the ciliary muscle relaxes which helps to alleviate pain. The patient must be informed and reassured about the loss of accommodation by the lens. It is best to avoid driving until the cornea has healed, which may take between 24 and 48 hours. Antibiotic prophylaxis helps to make the eye more comfortable (Marsden, 2002) especially in ointment form as the lubricant layer enables the lid to slide over the damaged epithelium. If the abrasions do not heal within 48–72 hours the patient must be referred to an ophthalmologist.

Recurrent corneal abrasion

Recurrent abrasion is a common complication of previous corneal abrasion. The epithelial cells fail to adhere to the basement membrane resulting in an unstable healing process. There is frequent loss of epithelium especially during rapid eye movements during sleep. The lid sticks to the loose cells which break when the patient opens their eyes after sleep. Many patients report waking up in the middle of the night with severe pain and foreign body sensation. During the daytime the pain is diminished because the damaged flap covers the abraded area. It is essential to prevent the condition occurring by using a bland ointment such as simple ointment at bedtime for 4 to 6 weeks. Patients are reassured by explaining to them the reasons for the pain occurring and how to prevent this from happening. Compliance is generally good.

Ultra violet light injury

UV radiation from welding or from sunlamps is absorbed by the surface corneal epithelium resulting in cell damage. Symptoms do not appear until 6–8 hours following exposure. This classically explains the midnight to 2am presentation of patients with what is often known as 'arc eye'. Arc eye is very painful as the nerves of the damaged epithelium are exposed. To alleviate the pain and patient distress one drop of local anaesthetic is instilled as per local protocol. On slit lamp examination and after instilled fluorescein dye the cornea shows multiple tiny staining spots known as Punctate Epithelial Erosions (PEE). Treatment involves prophylactic antibiotic and a lubricant ointment. Cycloplegic drops are at times prescribed. Oral analgesia is recommended for the first 12 hours. Health education to safeguard against future exposure to UV light is important, such as wearing visors. PEE heals within 24–48 hours.

Conjunctival abrasion and foreign body

Foreign bodies are a common occurrence on conjunctival surface. Marsden (2002) highlights that they rarely penetrate the conjunctiva and are therefore easily wiped off after instillation of local anaesthetic. The resulting, and any concurrent, abrasion, should be treated with an antibiotic ointment or drop. The patient will not require an eye pad as the degree of pain and discomfort is much less than with corneal injury.

Subtarsal foreign body (STFB)

The patient classically presents with a foreign body sensation underneath the upper eyelid which causes severe pain and watering during each blink. There may be a history of foreign body entering the eye but quite often the patient does not remember any such episode. With each blink the STFB causes superficial linear abrasions on the upper cornea which stains vividly with fluorescein dye. The upper lid is gently everted with a cotton bud for inspection and the foreign body wiped off with a sterile moistened swab. Once the STFB is removed the pain quickly disappears, thus there is no need to instil any local anaesthetic drops. Cheng *et al.* (1997) demonstrate that the patient can confirm when all the STFB has been removed. As corneal damage is superficial and minimal a single instillation of antibiotic drop or ointment is usually sufficient.

Corneal foreign body

Foreign bodies may enter the cornea during grinding, woodwork, brickwork etc. A superficial corneal foreign body is often easily removed with a moistened sterile cotton bud following instillation of topical anaesthetic. The resulting small abrasion is treated with antibiotic ointment. An embedded corneal foreign body is best removed using a slit lamp and a sterile hypodermic (usually 21 gauge) needle held tangentially to the cornea. The needle may be mounted on a cotton tipped swab or a syringe to aid removal.

After the initial removal of the foreign body, a rust ring often remains. The rust ring often dissipates with antibiotic ointment in a few days time. If it still persists the rust ring must be removed with care with a needle or dental burr.

Removal with a slit lamp provides adequate illumination and magnification with the patient's head well supported on the rest band. It is safer using a slit lamp as it also improves precision of the procedure, thus the risk of corneal perforation with the needle is eliminated. Following removal of the corneal foreign body, local anaesthetic is instilled and an eye pad applied for 24 hours. If the abrasion is small, i.e. less than 3 to 4 mm in diameter, some ophthalmologists would prefer not to pad the eye. The patient is instructed to take pain killers and rest at home for 24 hours. If the eye becomes red, painful and sticky with blurring of vision after the pad is removed the patient must seek ophthalmic advice immediately.

Serious closed eye injury

Bruising of the lids is an obvious sign of trauma to the eye and orbit which may be associated with ocular complications. Most 'black eyes' do not overlie an eye problem. It is important that an accurate visual acuity is obtained and the eye is examined.

Normal visual acuity indicates that ocular damage is minimal. If vision is disturbed, further ocular examination must take place and the patient should be referred to an ophthalmologist so that a thorough assessment can be carried out to identify the complication. A direct blow to the globe may damage all of the structures within it. The eye distorts with blunt injury, springs back into shape and tearing and bleeding of tissues within the eye may result. Secondary glaucoma from angle recession may result some months later.

A blunt trauma may tear the iris tissue and/or ciliary body resulting in blood in the anterior chamber (hyphaema). Traumatic hyphaema may be detectable only with a slit lamp (red blood cells floating in the anterior chamber) or may be visible with the naked eye as a reddish haze or a distinct level of blood inferiorly in the anterior chamber. Pain is very common and the pupil may be irregular or poorly reactive to light. All patients with hyphaema must be assessed by an ophthalmologist so that appropriate treatment can be given. Other injuries to the eye must be ruled out. If a patient with hyphaema needs to be transported, an upright position allows the red blood cells to settle in the anterior chamber thus clearing the visual axis so that the patient can see as much as possible. This may also help the patient to become less anxious and more co-operative.

Other intra-ocular complications following blunt severe trauma are given in Table 3.5.

Table 3.5

Intra-ocular complications of blunt trauma
Adapted from Marsden (2002)

Traumatic mydriasis	Damage to the iris sphincter muscles
Traumatic miosis	Spasm of the sphincter muscles associated with iritis.
Lens dislocation	Can be total or partial dislocation associated with blurred or uniocular diplopia
Damage to lens	Resulting in cataract which can occur rapidly
Retinal oedema (Commotio retinae)	Near the macula causing severe visual disturbance

Retinal haemorrhage or detachment	Flashing of lights, floaters, curtains floating over vision are suggestive of a detachment.
Raised intra-ocular pressure	Caused by hyphaema, inflammation or damage to the angle (angle recession); pain, photophobia and blurred vision are common symptoms.

The force of a blow can cause an orbital blow out fracture. The fracture occurs by transmission of force through the bones and soft tissues of the orbit by a non-penetrating object such as a fist or a ball. There is entrapment of muscles and orbital fat which reduces eye movement. Surgery is not always indicated as the symptoms often improve once the swelling subsides which tends to free the muscles and allow correct ocular motility.

Signs and symptoms include diplopia, enophthalmos, emphysema and infra-orbital anaesthesia, pain on eye movement and associated numbness of the lower cheek and upper lip depending where the fracture is. The infra-orbital nerve which is derived from the maxillary nerve may be involved if the maxillary bone is fractured. Blowing of the nose causes air from the nose to enter the orbital tissues and the lid to swell up with crepitus. Marsden (2002) points out that patients with orbital fractures and any visual disturbance should be referred early to an ophthalmologist. Meanwhile, patients are strongly advised not to blow their nose or strain at stool. Systemic antibiotics are prescribed to prevent orbital cellulitis. Patients are eventually referred to the orthoptist for monitoring of ocular movements and if within two weeks there is no improvement, surgical correction is carried out.

Orbital apex trauma is likely to cause optic nerve injury resulting in traumatic optic neuropathy. This can arise from both blunt trauma or from penetrating eye injury. There is a great risk of injury to the incoming cranial nerves in the orbit. When the 3rd, 4th and 6th cranial nerves are involved, extra-ocular palsy with diplopia will result. When the 5th cranial nerve is damaged, sensory disturbance to areas supplied by the trigeminal nerve will occur.

It is important to recognise the possibility of ocular involvement from indirect trauma such as base of skull fractures as well as more direct trauma where the eyes themselves do not appear to be involved. Patient complaints of loss of or reduction in vision must be taken very seriously and ophthalmological opinion obtained in order to stop preventable vision loss.

Retrobulbular haemorrhage may occur from blunt trauma to the orbit and progress rapidly resulting in pain, proptosis, lid and conjunctival swelling and engorged conjunctival vessels. Subconjunctival haemorrhage may be present. If the eye begins to protrude after trauma an ophthalmologist should be seen immediately. CT or MRI scan may be required urgently and the patient's visual acuity should be checked very frequently, probably every 15 minutes. If vision deteriorates, emergency decompression of the haemorrhage by lateral canthotomy under local anaesthetic will be required to relieve pressure on the optic nerve.

Open trauma

An open eye injury requires prompt ophthalmic assessment. If there are any retained materials protruding from the eye no attempt should be made to remove them. The material should be stabilised as far as possible perhaps by taping it to the cheek if this seems appropriate or by covering the whole area with a plastic shield.

No pressure should be applied on to an eye with a full thickness injury and while it might be appropriate to cover the area with a pad, this should be done with care. The pad must be loose and taped well away from the globe. Patients with even very severe eye trauma may not have much pain if there is little corneal epithelial loss. The control of any pain and nausea must be a priority as vomiting is likely to lead to loss of ocular contents. To minimise any increase in intra-ocular pressure, Marsden (2002) advocates that the patient must be lying flat or sitting up at around a 30 degree angle.

Lid laceration must also be dealt with immediately. Full lid laceration may also involve the globe and all due care must be taken to avoid firm pressure on the globe. It is important to rule out globe involvement by recording visual acuity and careful assessment of the globe using the slit lamp.

Repair of lid trauma may be delayed due to the extremely good vascularisation of the lids and associated structures and may therefore be a planned activity rather than an emergency one, leading to the best possible functional and cosmetic result for the patient.

Both penetrating and non-penetrating eye injuries require careful and thorough assessment. With appropriate management many patients have a very good chance of retaining useful vision. Accurate recording of visual acuity and documentation of care are essential for medico-legal reasons.

Ocular trauma in children

Eye injuries are a leading cause of visual impairment and monocular blindness in children (Kutschke, 1994). De Respinis *et al.* (1989) state that the frequency of eye injuries in children is high and at least 90% of all eye injuries to children could be prevented. This is more common in boys than girls, in a ratio of 3:1 according to Kutsche (1994). This presumably occurs because of the highly physical contact among and more aggressive nature of boys.

Older children and adolescents show a higher incidence of trauma than infants or toddlers (Rapoport *et al.*, 1990). This increase in eye trauma is probably the result of more unsupervised play among older children. This tends to occur more during spring and summer months when warm weather provides the opportunity for outdoor play. In contrast, Niranen and Raivio (1981) found that in Finland the commonest cause of ocular injury was snowballs.

Possible causes of eye injuries are everywhere – at home, school and play. Nelson *et al.* (1989) state that no place is totally safe. Within the home, almost anything is a potential trauma cause. Sharp items such as knives, forks, scissors, furniture edges and household chemicals can all cause serious eye injury. Toys are a major source of eye injury. Kutschke (1994) found that products that caused the injuries ranged from crayons to toy guns. At the top of the list was bicycles and BB pellets and air guns. Although BB guns are labelled as suitable for children as young as 8 years old they should never be considered toys. Nelson *et al.* (1989) state that these guns are the leading cause of perforating injuries and subsequent enucleation in children. The group at greatest risk for BB gun related injuries is between 5 and 14 years, boys comprising 80–90% according to Grin *et al.* (1987). Sports and recreation are another major cause of ocular trauma. Kutschke (1994) highlights that hospital emergency departments treated

39,526 eye injuries caused by sports and recreational products in 1991. Ball sports, swimming, baseball, basketball and football largely account for these injuries.

Nelson *et al.* (1989) found that there is poor compliance with protective eyewear among young children when paying baseball, consequently baseball is the main cause of sports related eye injuries in the USA. Elman (1986) found that many players refuse to wear proper protective eyewear despite the compelling data supporting its use. The attitude that 'it can't happen to me' foolishly courts disaster. Many amateurs irrationally refuse to wear protective devices because they claim that it takes away 'the edge' from their game. This transient 'edge' frequently is bought at the expense of permanent and severe visual disability. Elman (1986) stresses that preventive medicine must form the cornerstone of trauma management regardless of the cause. Therefore anyone who participates in sports should wear eye protection. Kutschke (1994) points out if it is not mandated by the rules committee of that sport, it should be strongly suggested by the ophthalmic professional and parents. Anyone who is 'one eyed' must wear safety glasses at all times to protect the remaining eye. This also applies to amblyopes as they have a higher risk of becoming blind than the general population.

Ocular trauma in children varies from mild bruising with no loss of vision to rupture of the globe and permanent loss of vision. The health professional must take an accurate history from the child and parents and keep documentation of visual acuity for medico-legal reasons. All children who sustain an eye injury must be referred to an ophthalmologist for a thorough ophthalmic assessment so that appropriate care can be given to save sight.

Virtually any childhood ocular trauma condition can occur as a result of abuse or neglect (Taylor and Hoyt, 1997). The healthcare worker should be alerted when discrepancies are suggested or the nature of the injury is incompatible with the care providers' history of events. Child abuse (non-accidental injury) affecting the eye may take many forms according to the Ophthalmology Child Abuse Working Party (1999). The form most commonly encountered by a paediatric ophthalmologist is that associated with intra-cerebral injury and results from severe shaking, with or without additional impact injury. Extensive retinal haemorrhage has been regarded as a marker for 'shaken baby syndrome'. There are various distinct forms of child abuse, many of which may involve the visual system:

a. Physical abuse
   Indirect trauma and shaking
   Direct eye trauma
   Smothering
   Poisoning

b. Induced illness: Munchausen Syndrome by Proxy

c. Sexual abuse

d. Neglect

e. Emotional abuse.

Unilateral retinal haemorrhage exceeding 20–30% of the total retinal area must be regarded as a very strong indicator for violent shaking according to Betz *et al.* (1996).

The implications of child abuse are covered in Chapter 6. Child abuse is a complex issue and its effects on the eye and brain result in a complex interplay of social, legal, clinical biomechanical and pathological factors.

Considerable force is needed to produce a retinal or brain injury even if a shaking injury is non-accidental. This does not necessarily imply that the resulting injuries are the effect intended by the assailant. There may be further need for campaigns that draw parents' and other carers' attention to the fact that the effects of shaking may be more severe than expected.

Prevention of childhood eye injuries is extremely important. Parents should do the following:

- childproof the home and supervise children's activities
- enforce the use of protective eyewear during sports activities
- educate the child not to treat missiles, projectile air or BB guns as toys.

Ophthalmic professionals and associated health professionals should do the following:

- advise parents of the advantages of polycarbonate spectacles for all children
- emphasise the role of spectacles as a protective device to parents
- document patient discussion regarding eye safety in records and

- follow-up on compliance with safety glasses wear (i.e. question patients specifically at follow up visits, document patients' responses in patient records).

Most accidental childhood eye injuries are preventable. Adherence to these guidelines could significantly reduce the number and severity of these injuries. This is reinforced by Stevens (1998) who states that health promotion to prevent eye injuries can be achieved by raising community awareness and involvement. It is a challenge to all health workers who may, consequently, make a significant contribution to the prevention of eye injuries. Prevention must be at the core of eye injury management, whatever the cause.

THINKING POINT

TAKE A FEW MINUTES TO REFLECT ON HOW YOU WOULD PROVIDE HEALTH PROMOTION AND SUPPORT IN THE FOLLOWING SITUATIONS:

- A patient has sustained a traumatic corneal abrasion while gardening
- A young apprentice builder accidentally splashes wet cement into both eyes while at work
- A 5-year-old boy has sustained a bruise and laceration to his right upper lid from colliding with the sharp corner of a table while playing with his two older brothers at home. He is accompanied by his parent.

Patient decision-making and the use of the Health Belief Model

The Health Belief Model

Millions of people each year attend Accident and Emergency departments (Walsh, 1995). The number of attendances has steadily grown during the past few years (Blythin, 1988). There has been much debate about the use made by the general public of Accident and Emergency services according to Walsh (1995). Walsh (1995) explores the notion of the Health Belief Model which predicts that individuals carry out a treatment cost-benefit analysis when making decisions about seeking medical assistance. Sbaih (1993) showed that many patients are seen as 'rule breakers' or 'inappropriate attenders but she stresses the need to consider the patient's perceptions before arriving at such judgemental labels.

Medical research into A&E usage by Davison *et al.* (1983) showed that 39% of a sample of 587 A&E patients were neither accident nor emergency cases, according to the clinical judgement of the casualty officers and therefore should not be seen in an A&E department. Furthermore Myers (1982) claimed that 54% of a sample of 1000 A&E patients could be dealt with by a general practitioner. Walsh (1995) discusses the significance of attribution theory that offers some explanation in that staff may be making attributions to patients in connection with their attendance that are internal in nature rather than external. External attribution refers to justification made by a person about the factors affecting their life, which make it more logical for them to attend A&E, rather than their GP surgery. For instance the patients assess their susceptibility to ill health, the risk involved, the cost and likely benefits of treatment before deciding to seek medical help. This suggests that the patients make a cost-benefit analysis and will decide to attend A&E if the perceived benefits outweigh the perceived costs.

Internal attribution theory applies to staff getting into stigmatisation and blaming patients for non-attendance or for non-compliance, leading to victim blaming. External attribution might be concerning the quality of health care they will be getting, e.g. if members of their family had previously suffered harm in the hospital, the patients might think very carefully before attending for treatment.

This tendency to ignore outside factors and see only the person as responsible for their behaviour has been termed the 'fundamental attribution error' by Ross (1977), indicating the importance of this error in perception. Attribution theory would therefore suggest that A&E staff may ignore the possibility that there are sound reasons affecting the person's everyday life which make it logical for them to present to A&E rather than their GP. Instead, the patient is held responsible for their attendance and an internal attribution is made.

Helman (1991) points out that the perceptions of illness held by the public and health professionals are usually different, particularly with regard to the significance of symptoms. This insight indicates that the general public may well behave in ways that seem inappropriate to health professionals when confronted by illness and injury.

Many patients with an ophthalmic disorder will prefer to attend an A&E department. This supports the evidence put forward by Wood and Cliff (1986) who found that a common patient perception was the A&E was better or quicker than the GP. A further key theory that explains attendance patterns is the Health Belief Model (Rosenstock 1974). This proposes that individuals assess their susceptibility to ill health, the risks involved, the costs and likely benefits of treatment before deciding to seek medical help. This suggests that the patient makes a cost-benefit analysis and will decide to attend A&E if the perceived benefits outweigh the perceived costs. Many patients with ocular pain and visual disturbance will much prefer not to waste time at the GP surgery and will attend A&E having made a cost-benefit analysis. Jones *et al.* (1991) support the application of the Health Belief Model to the A&E field with their work showing improvements in compliance amongst patients treated in the emergency department.

The work of Mechanic (1992) also addresses reasons to seek medical help and these include seriousness of symptoms, disruption of everyday life and competing needs, accessibility of treatment and the pain and anxiety generated by the condition. Again, there are strong elements of cost and threat being weighed against the benefits of treatment in this approach. A typical ophthalmic condition is an acute iridocyclitis associated with severe ocular pain, blurring of vision, photophobia, watering and redness. This will have severe implications for sight if left untreated or if mismanaged by the GP with local antibiotics. Ophthalmic management in this instance is vital to save sight and to prevent secondary ocular complications such as cataract, glaucoma and pan uveitis.

The patient must be assessed by an expert practitioner and evaluated within 5 minutes of their arrival in the A&E department to keep in line with government initiatives (DoH 1995). Practitioners in the Accident and Emergency department need to be able to identify those patients whose needs are urgent.

Accident and Emergency attendance therefore needs to be seen as a result of logical decision-making processes that requires hospitals to provide appropriate services, rather than merely labelling the patient as inappropriate.

THINKING POINT

TAKE A FEW MINUTES TO READ THIS SCENARIO FROM PRACTICE AND THEN DISCUSS IT WITH A WORK COLLEAGUE.

Ibrahim Shah is a 35-year-old city banker who suffers from chronic eczema, asthma and chronic scalp dandruff. His eyes often become sore and uncomfortable with blurred vision, at times sticky on waking up and occasionally he is photo-phobic.

His visual acuities are 6/12 in each eye unaided and improve to 6/6 with pinhole occluder. He works at a famous bank and does not like taking time off to see his doctor. Today he attends the A&E department because his symptoms seem much worse than previously.

Discuss the appropriateness of his attendance to the Accident and Emergency department. Debate your points with your colleague to support his decision to attend.

Conclusion

This chapter has explored the challenging issues around ophthalmic emergencies and the care and management of patients in the Accident and Emergency department. What constitutes effective triage management was discussed alongside the need for practitioners to have a sound knowledge and understanding of the application of the law and ethics to professional practice. In particular, it was stressed that children with eye problems must be given due attention from the outset.

The management of ophthalmic emergencies requires prioritisation and immediate appropriate action in order to salvage sight. It also highlights that effective teamwork and communication within a triage system promote safer care.

References

Alcock, D., Goodman, J.T., Feldman, W., and McGrath, P.J. (1985). 'Environment and waiting behaviour in emergency rooms.' *Children's Health Care* 13 (4): 174–80.

Banerjee, S., Beatty, S., Tyagi, A., and Kirkby, G.R. (1998). 'The role of ophthalmic triage and the nurse practitioner in an eye dedicated casualty department.' *Eye* 12: 880–2.

Bentley, J. (1995). 'Triage of children in A&E: research shortfall addressed.' *Nursing Times* 91 (51): 38–9.

Betz, P., Eisenmenger, W., Lignitz, E., Miltner, E., and Puschel, K. (1996). 'Morphometrical analysis of retinal haemorrhages in the shaken baby syndrome.' *Forensic Science International* 78: 71–80.

Bickerton, R. (2000). 'Identifying and treating ocular emergencies.' *Journal of Ophthalmic Nursing and Technology* 19 (5): 225–9.

Blythin, P. (1998). Triage in the UK. *Nursing* 3 (31): 16–20.

Buchan, J.C., Saihan, Z., and Reynolds, A.G. (2003). 'Nurse triage, diagnosis and treatment of eye casualty patients: a study of quality and utility.' *Accident and Emergency Nursing* 11 (4): 226–8.

Burlew, A. (1991). 'Preventing eye injuries – The nurse's role.' *Insight The Journal of the American Society of Ophthalmic Registered Nurses* 24 (6): 24–8.

Cheng, H., Burdon, M.A., Buckley, S.A., and Moorman, C. (1997). *Emergency Ophthalmology.* London: BMJ Publishing Group.

Cioffi, J. (1999). 'Triage decision-making: Educational strategies.' Accident and Emergency Nursing 7: 106–11.

Crouch, R. (1994). 'Triage: past, present and future.' Emergency Nurse 2: 4–6.

Davey, C.C. (1996). 'The red eye.' *British Journal of Hospital Medicine* 55 (3): 89–94.

Davis, A.R., and Ali, Q.H. (1997). 'Topical steroid use in the treatment of ocular alkali burns.' *British Journal of Ophthalmology* 81: 732–4.

Davison, A., Hildrey, A., and Floyer, M. (1983). 'Use and misuses of an A&E Department in the East End of London.' *Journal of the Royal Society of Medicine* 76: 37–40.

Department of Health (1991). *The Welfare of Children and Young People in Hospital.* London: HMSO.

Department of Health (1995). *The Patients' Charter and You.* London: HMSO.

Department of Health (2004). *The National Service Framework for Children, Young People and Maternity Services.* London: HMSO. www.actionforsickchildren.org (last accessed 2.6.09).

De Respinis, P.A., Caputo, A.R., and Fiore, P.M. (1989). 'A survey of severe eye injuries in children.' *American Journal of Diseases of Children* 143: 711–16.

Duffy, B. (2008). 'Managing chemical eye injuries.' *Emergency Nurse* 16 (1): 25–9.

Duguid, G. (1997). 'Red eye: avoid the pitfalls.' *The Practitioner* 241: 188–95.

Elman, M.J. (1986). 'Racket sports ocular injuries.' *Archives of Ophthalmology* 104: 1453–4.

Falcon, M. (1989). *Supplement to Mims Magazine*. Aylesbury: Leo Laboratories Ltd.

Forrester, J., Dick, A., McMenamin, P., and Lee, W. (1996). *The Eye: Basic Sciences in Practice*. London: Saunders.

Glenn, S. (1995). 'Care of patients with chemical eye injury.' *Emergency Nurse* 3: 3.

Grin, T.R., Nelson, L.B., and Jeffers, J.B. (1987). 'Eye injuries in childhood.' *Paediatrics* 80: 13–17.

Health and Safety Executive (2001). *HSE Safety and Enforcement Statistics*. Merseyside: Statistical Services Unit.

Helman, C. (1991). *Culture, Health and Illness*. Oxford: Butterworth-Heinemann.

Hooper, M. (1997). 'Prompt treatment for chemical eye injuries.' *Nursing Standard* 11: 40–43.

Jatla, K.K., and Zhao, F. (2008). 'Conjunctivitis' *Neonatal e-Medicine*, updated 17 November 2008.
Available at: http://emedicine.medscape.com/article/1192190-overview.

Jones, G. (1988). 'Top priority.' *Nursing Standard* 3 (7): 28–9.

Jones, S., Jones, P., and Katz, J. (1991). 'Compliance in acute and chronic patients receiving a health belief model intervention in the emergency department.' *Social Science of Medicine* 32 (10): 1183–9.

Judge, J. (1992). 'Overview of the red eye.' *Journal of Ophthalmic Nursing and Technology* 11 (5): 197–202.

Kutschke, P. J. (1994). 'Ocular trauma in children.' *Journal of Ophthalmic Nursing & Technology* 13 (3): 117–19.

MacCumber, M.W. (1998). *The Management of Ocular Injuries and Emergencies*. Philadelphia: Lippincott Raven Publishers.

McDonald, L., Butterworth, T., and Yates, D.W. (1995). 'Triage: a literature review 1985—1993.' *Accident and Emergency Nursing* 3: 201–7.

MacEwen, C. J. (1989). 'Eye injuries: a prospective survey of 5671 cases.' *British Journal of Ophthalmology* 73: 888–94.

McGrory, A. (1996). 'Eye injuries: a review of the literature with nursing implications.' *International Journal of Nursing Studies* 34 (2): 87–92.

Marsden, J. (1999). 'Expert nurse decision-making: Telephone triage in an ophthalmic accident and emergency department.' *Nursing Times Research* 4 (1): 44–54.

Marsden, J. (2002). 'Ophthalmic trauma in the Accident and Emergency Department.' *Accident and Emergency Nursing* 10: 136–42.

Mechanic, D. (1992). 'Health & illness behaviour and patient/practitioner relationships.' *Social Science of Medicine* 34 (12): 1345–50.

Milligan, H. (2002). 'The aetiology of ocular trauma and the ophthalmic nurse's role in its prevention.' *Ophthalmic Nursing* 5 (4): 14–18.

Murray, W.F. (1988). 'Epidemic keratoconjunctivitis.' *Annals of Ophthalmology* 20: 36–8.

Myers, P. (1982). 'Management of minor medical problems and trauma: general practice or hospital?' *Journal of the Royal Society of Medicine* 75: 879–83.

Nelson, L.B., Wilson, T.W., and Jeffers, J.B. (1989). 'Eye injuries in childhood:

Demography, etiology and prevention.' *Paediatrics* **84**: 438–41.

Niranen, M., and Raivio, I. (1981). 'Eye injuries in children.' *British Journal of Ophthalmology* 65: 436–8.

O'Driscoll, A.M., Shah, P., Aggrawal, R.K., Chell, P.B., Hope-Ross, M.W., and McDonnell, P.J. (1995). 'Ocular injuries due to alkaline substances.' *British Medical Journal* 310: 943.

Ophthalmology Child Abuse Working Party (1999). 'Child abuse and the eye.' *Eye, Royal College of Ophthalmologists*, 13: 3–10.

Parmar, M., and Hewitt, E. (1985). 'Triage on trial.' *Senior Nurse* 2 (5): 21–2.

Pau, H. (1978). *Differential Diagnosis of Eye Diseases*. Philadelphia: Saunders.

Phillips, B.M., and Robson, W.J. (1992). 'Paediatrics in the accident and emergency department.' *Archives of Disease in Childhood* 67: 560–4.

Randleman, J.B. (2006). 'Chemical burns.' *e-Medicine*, updated 22 September 2006.

Rapoport, I., Romem, M., and Kinek, M. (1990). 'Eye injuries in children in Israel: A nationwide collaborative study.' *Archives of Ophthalmology* 108: 376–9.

Roper-Hall, M.J. (1965). 'Thermal and chemical burns of the eye.' *Transactions of the Ophthalmological Societies of the UK* 85: 631–46.

Rosenstock, I. (1974). 'Historical origins of the health belief model.' *Health Education Monographs* 2: 328–35.

Ross, L. (1977). 'The intuitive psychologist and his shortcomings: distortions in the attribution process.' In Berkowitz, I. ed. *Advances in Experimental Social Psychology*, Vol. 10. New York: Academic Press.

Sbaih, L. (1993). 'Accident and emergency work, a review of some of the literature.' *Journal of Advanced Nursing* 18: 957–62.

Schmidt, E.R., and Kramer, J. (1997). 'Consumer product related eye injuries.' *Journal of Ophthalmic Nursing and Technology* 16 (5): 251–5.

Seewoodhary, M. (1983). 'Common presentations in accident and emergency.' *Nursing, the add-on Journal of Clinical Nursing* 2 (17): 498–500.

Seewoodhary, R. (2003). 'Subconjunctival haemorrhage: implications for ophthalmic nursing practice.' *Ophthalmic Nursing* 7: 10–14.

Stevens, S. (1998). 'Eye injuries: Causes and prevention.' *Ophthalmic Nursing* 2 (3): 25–31.

Stetson, N.G. (1986). 'Telephone triage in the ambulatory care setting.' *Journal of Ophthalmic Nursing and Technology* 5 (6): 219–22.

Taylor, D., and Hoyt, C. (1997). *Practical Paediatric Ophthalmology*. Oxford: Blackwell Science.

Thompson, C., Dowding, D., and McCaughan, D. (2004). 'Strategies for avoiding pitfalls in clinical decision making.' *Nursing Times* 100 (20): 40–2.

Walsh, M. (1995). 'The health belief model and use of accident and emergency services by the general public.' *Journal of Advanced Nursing* 22: 694–9.

Wilson, R. J. (1986). 'Subconjunctival haemorrhage overview and management.' *Journal of American Optometric Association* 57 (5): 376–80.

Wood, T., and Cliff, K. (1986). 'AE departments: why people attend with minor injuries and ailments.' *Public Health* 100: 15–20.

York, S., and Proud, G. (1990). 'Ophthalmic triage.' *Nursing Times* 86: 8.

Chapter 4
Managing contact lenses and associated eye problems
Ramesh Seewoodhary

Background
Classification of soft contact lenses
Associated eye problems
Patient compliance
The fitting of contact lenses and current legislation

Introduction

Chapter 3 has provided an insight into ophthalmic triage, decision-making, the red eye, eye injuries and the Health Belief Model. Many of the issues discussed in this chapter are also applicable to patients with contact lens problems. Red eyes, conjunctivitis, and corneal injury are all problems which may be presented by contact lens wearers. In most cases, the contact lens patients would need to attend an ophthalmic outpatient department for management of their eye complications, which mostly arise from overuse, or allergic reactions.

Chapter 4 commences with a discussion of the background to contact lens care and provides a short history of contact lenses. Associated eye problems are presented and discussed with reference to some of the current challenges such as patient compliance and current legislation related to the fitting of contact lenses (Optician's Act, 1989). Importantly, one of the most devastating complications of contact lens wear, Acanthamoeba keratitis, is addressed. Hygiene is one of the most important factors to consider in the effective management of contact lens wearers.

Background

Background

Since their introduction in the mid-1970s, hydrophilic soft contact lenses have been an important part of the ophthalmologist's toolkit for the treatment of corneal and external diseases, as well as for the correction of refractive errors. Despite the great value of soft contact lenses, the most serious contact lens related complication is bacterial keratitis (Stern, 1998). It has taken ophthalmic scientists nearly 20 years of clinical experience and laboratory investigation to gain a comprehensive knowledge of why soft contact lens wearers develop corneal infections.

More than 3 million people in the UK wear contact lenses and the number of wearers is increasing annually (Dart, 1993). 97% of people wearing contact lenses do so for correction of refractive errors (Schein *et al.*, 1989). Contact lenses are popular for reasons of convenience, efficiency in aiding vision for certain sports and occupations and for their cosmetic advantage (Polse, 1991). The rise in contact lens wear has increased the number of people at risk of contact lens related complications. Moore (1990) states that education of the contact lens wearer is the key to the prevention of complications. People who wear soft contact lenses overnight are 15 times more likely to develop a sight threatening infection than those using the most up-to-date rigid lenses (Ferriman, 1991). The classification of soft contact lenses is given in Table 4.1.

Table 4.1

The classification of soft contact lenses
Adapted from Stern (1998)

Therapeutic bandage contact lenses	Useful in treatment of: • Bullous keratopathy • Filamentary keratitis • Persistent epithelial defects • Sealing of small corneal perforations High risk of infection in patients with ocular surface diseases
Daily wear cosmetic soft contact lenses	Used for optical purposes for daytime wear only. Poor compliance with hygiene regime leading to gram negative corneal infection, by *Pseudomonas aeruginosa*

Extended wear cosmetic lenses	Used for optical purposes including overnight wear.
	Carry a higher risk of microbial keratitis than other types of lenses.
Disposable soft contact lenses	Used for optical purposes
	More expensive than non-disposable lenses
	Non-compliance is a problem and patients can develop bacterial keratitis.

Associated eye problems

Associated eye problems

Epithelial defect provides a site for bacteria to adhere to the cornea at its leading injured edge (Stern, 1990). Once the bacteria adhere to the injured epithelium they rapidly reach the stromal layer by a process of trans-epithelial migration. Reichert and Stern (1984) found that the most common causes of corneal ulceration are *Pseudomonas aeruginosa, Staphylococcus aureus* and *Streptococci pneumoniae*. They adhere well to the human corneal epithelium. The adherence process is facilitated by both pili and lipopolysaccharides in gram negative bacteria.

Many contact lens patients who develop bacterial keratitis do not take proper care of their lenses. The disinfectant and the storage case frequently become contaminated (Stern, 1998). Over 50% of contaminated cases contain pseudomonas and other gram negative bacilli. Pseudomonas readily adheres to the plastic surface of cases where the adherent organisms secrete a slime that enables them to survive disinfecting solutions. Contact lenses stored in such cases quickly become contaminated.

Contact lenses quickly become coated with tear film on insertion. The tear film contains mucin and protein which are good breeding grounds for bacteria. Sialic acid, an important receptor for Pseudomonas, is a component of mucin which can enhance adherence of Pseudomonas to worn lenses. Once bacteria adhere to lenses the production of organic biofilm further strengthens the attachment (Miller and Ahearn, 1987). The average worn lens harbours over 2,000 bacteria and may carry up to 150,000 organisms (Mowrey-Mckee *et al.*, 1992). Figure 4.1

shows a hydrophilic contact lens with mucoprotein lipid deposition.

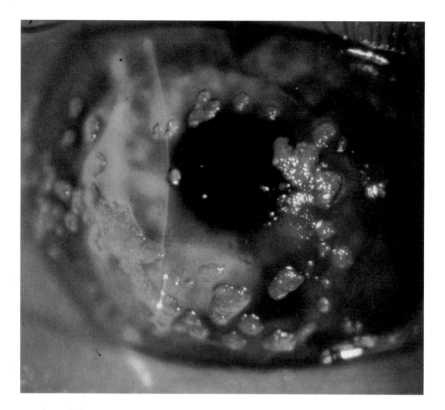

Figure 4.1

Hydrophilic contact lens with mucoprotein lipid deposition
With kind permission of Moorfields Eye Hospital Medical Photography Department

Hypoxia of lens wear causes chronic partial desquamation of the epithelial surface, creating sites for bacteria to adhere. This is aggravated by the overnight wear of contact lenses. The bacteria can easily invade the stromal layer of the cornea. During the process of invasion the lens further impedes the influx of white blood cells allowing for a period of unchecked bacterial replication. When the white blood cells do reach the stroma, the clinical signs of a bacterial corneal ulcer occur. In future it is anticipated that scientists will create a cost-competitive disposable daily wear lens with better oxygen transmissibility and with surface modifications to inhibit the development of coatings and resist the adherence of bacteria.

Satisfying the oxygen demands of the eye is critical for long-term success with contact lenses. Several factors affect the oxygen transmissibility of a contact lens according to Rakow (1999). These include the permeability of the lens material, the average thickness of the lens, the temperature of the eye and the amount of lens movement which affects the amount of oxygen supplied through the tear pump. Tear exchange upon blinking is negligible in soft lens wearers. Depending on the lens design the lid can deliver as much as one-third of the oxygen necessary to avoid corneal oedema in rigid lens wearers.

Some of the complications of contact lens wear as identified by Rakow (1999) are given in Table 4.2.

Table 4.2

Complications of contact lens wear Adapted from Rakow (1999)

	Definition
a. Superficial punctuate keratitis	Desquamation of superficial epithelial cells
b. Stromal oedema and vertical striae	Swelling of stromal layer caused by a break in the epithelium or endothelium barriers. Striae may be seen in the Descemet's layer
c. Spectacle blur	Blurring of vision with glasses after lens removal caused by concomitant corneal steepening and irregularity.
d. Oedematous corneal formations	These are branching lesions in the central epithelium that are seen most often in Polymethyl methacrylate (PMMA) lens wearers. They are hypoxic in origin and may persist for months.
e. Over-wearing syndrome	Over-wear of PMMA rigid lenses, erratic wearing schedules or failure to follow the recommended wearing schedule during lens adaptation or re-adaptation may result in over-wearing abrasions.
f. Decreased corneal sensitivity	Corneal hypoxia can result in a marked decrease in corneal sensitivity due to damage to corneal nerve endings.
g. Corneal exhaustion syndrome	Corneal oedema that tends to occur after 6–8 hours of contact lens wear with recurrent corneal abrasions, loss of corneal lustre, an increase in lens discomfort and gradual loss of tolerance.

continued overleaf

h. Myopia creep	Soft lens induced hypoxia causes corneal oedema. This is accompanied by a gradual increase in myopia.
i. Neovascularisation	New vessels on the corneal surface caused by hypoxia.
j. Corneal infiltrates	Clumped up white blood cells and lymphocytes – these occur as discrete circular lesions in the mid peripheral cornea. They may be hypoxic in origin or result from infection or solution sensitivity.
k. Acute red-eye syndrome	Red eye caused by hypoxia which is painful. Photophobia and tearing are present. Epithelial staining may be present as well as sub-epithelial or anterior or stromal infiltrates near the limbal area.
l. Epithelial sloughing	Prolonged hypoxia in soft lens wearers can result in 80 % loss of corneal epithelium, accompanied by severe pain and photophobia.

Sight threatening corneal infection by Acanthamoeba is the most severe complication arising from contact lens wear. Acanthamoeba is a living protozoon and is found in contaminated water, e.g. swimming pools, hot tubs, tap water, distilled water used to prepare homemade saline. It invades the damaged corneal epithelium progressing to the stromal layer where it feeds on the corneal keratocytes.

The appearance of Acanthamoeba keratitis differs in early disease (Dart 1995). Familiarity with the early signs of the disease is important because the clinical features of the infection are seldom shared with corneal infections due to other micro-organisms. Appropriate treatment in early disease results in a medical cure, with minimal visual loss, in a high proportion of patients. Late disease has a poor prognosis due to scar tissue formation, and intra-ocular complications.

In the early disease the typical features are punctate keratopathy, pseudo dendrites, epithelial infiltrates, diffuse and focal subepithelial infiltrates and radial keratoneuritis. Although radial keratoneuritis has been reported in association with other causes of corneal infection it is almost diagnostic for Acanthamoeba keratitis. Epithelial defects are relatively uncommon in early disease. Limbitis and anterior scleritis are common early features and may be associated with severe pain. Acanthamoeba keratitis is often associated with ring infiltrates and corneal ulceration, which is sometimes indolent and sometimes relapsing. These are typical signs of late disease and rarely seen within four weeks of the onset of symptoms. Figure 4.2 shows the characteristic features of Acanthamoeba keratitis.

Polymicrobial infection with bacteria has been reported in up to 10% of cases and may be more common. Simultaneous infection with bacteria may account for the presence of early focal ulceration and a ring abscess complicating the clinical picture in early Acanthamoeba keratitis. Similarly in late disease, bacterial super-infection is common. These possibilities must be considered if the clinical course alters.

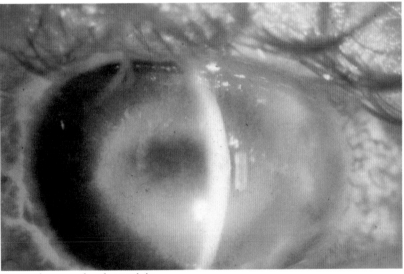

Figure 4.2

Acanthamoeba keratitis
With kind permission of Moorfields Eye Hospital Medical Photography Department

Medical treatment of Acanthamoeba keratitis has been shown by Dart (1995) to be effective in cases treated within one month of the onset of symptoms. Unfortunately the diagnosis is often delayed by several months because of mis-diagnosis as Herpes simplex virus keratitis, resulting in advanced disease, refractory to treatment (Bacon *et al.*, 1993). Medical treatment is difficult to manage. Effective amoebicidal drugs are few and many have toxic side effects on the corneal epithelium. Bacterial super-infection of established ulcers is common and may be mistreated as a reactivation of amoebic infection. Several anti-fungals, antibiotics and antiseptics have been shown to be effective against trophozoites but it is probable that it is the effect against the more resistant encysted form of Acanthamoeba that determines the success or failure of treatment. The prevention of Acanthamoeba keratitis in both established and emerging markets requires patient and practitioner education regarding the risks of poor compliance with lens hygiene as well as the development of improved and simplified disinfection methods for Acanthamoeba and bacteria.

New lens systems such as the daily disposable soft lens have the potential for reducing the incidence to much lower levels. The incidence of the disease is approximately 1 in 20,000 contact lens wearers per year (Seal and Kirkness, 1995). As contact lens wear increases there appears to be an increase in Acanthamoeba keratitis. Such infection can be devastating with prolonged morbidity if untreated or if non-acanthamoebicidal drugs are used. Laboratory confirmation is vital as medical misjudgements can occur. This is primarily due to the similarity in clinical presentation to that of Herpes simplex keratitis. Early recognition can be successfully treated according to Bacon *et al.*, (1993). The storage case must be kept in a clean uncontaminated state to prevent microbial growth. The case must be rinsed daily in boiled, cooled water at 70°C from a domestic kettle and dried by inversion on to absorbent paper. Water taken directly from a tap should never be used as part of contact lens hygiene practice. The case must be stored dry until next used. This simple, but effective, procedure will prevent pathogens infecting the lens storage case.

Patient compliance

Patient compliance

Optimal hygiene practice is vital as a preventative measure against microbial keratitis including that due to Acanthamoeba. Compliance with contact lens care regimen is the key to preventing lens-induced complications yet many studies show that as many as 70% of all contact lens wearers are non-compliant in one or more aspects of a care regimen (Rakow, 1993). Patients may fail to use a disinfection system appropriate for their type of lenses, may fail to follow the recommended frequency of routine lens care, or may fail to clean and disinfect their lenses. Some patients slowly lapse into non-compliance and begin to skip steps; others follow the prescribed steps in the wrong order or add steps in the wrong places.

There is a tendency to shorten the recommended disinfection time and a failure by even the most meticulous patients to keep their lens cases clean. Some patients begin to sleep in lenses that are old, discoloured or badly coated. Some patients are tempted by sales and purchase products not recommended for their eyes or for their lenses. Products are often used beyond their expiry dates or are subjected to improper handling and contamination. This may occur if solution bottles are left uncovered or if the tips of bottles are touched to the eyes, lashes, lenses or skin. Some patients fail to understand the purpose of a disinfecting solution and store their lenses in nothing but saline at night. Many patients neglect proper lens care because of laziness, fatigue late in the evening when lenses should be cleaned and disinfected, or expense. They may not have understood the instructions given at the dispensing visit, particularly if they are very young, very old, have difficulty with the English language or they may have failed to receive adequate instruction.

Poor hand hygiene may result in the transfer of bacteria, fungi, cosmetics, creams or nicotine from the wearer to the lenses. Surfactant cleaners, combined with friction, remove 90–95% of the micro-organisms from the lens surface and increase the efficiency of the disinfecting solution. Deposits that are not removed can lead to poor visual acuity, red eyes, giant papillary conjunctivitis, corneal staining and oedema and reduced lens life.

The weakness of a lens care system may be traced to the patient, the practitioner or the technician. Systems that are too expensive, too complex or too inconvenient may encourage shortcuts and result in serious eye complications.

People learn best by doing therefore the technician must show the steps involved in lens care and then ask the patient to perform each step. It should not be assumed that patients who have worn lenses before are caring for them properly. They too should receive full care instructions and be asked to run through them in proper sequence. Each patient must be given not only verbal instructions, but also written instructions to be kept for permanent reference. At follow-up visits patients should be asked to relate or demonstrate exactly what they do when they take their lenses out each night. Any lapses in compliance or misunderstandings should be noted and proper care reviewed. Phone calls to clarify questions should be encouraged. Patients must be told never to borrow solutions from friends or to buy solutions that have not been specifically recommended for their lenses or their eyes without first consulting with their eye care practitioner. If patients understand that contact lenses are not just another vision correcting modality but medical devices that should be worn in the eyes under carefully controlled conditions they will be more likely to comply. An educated patient is the best insurance against contact lens induced complications. Patients must always adopt a positive attitude towards understanding a proper lens care regime and be motivated to do so at all times if they are to be risk free.

Everyone has a different lifestyle and to reflect this, there are different wearing schedules for contact lenses as shown in Table 4.3.

Table 4.3

Contact lenses at a glance

Source: British Contact Lens Association (BCLA).Taken from http://www.bcla.org.uk/wearing_schedules.asp (accessed on 13 February 2006).

	Soft (Disposable)	Soft (Traditional)	Soft (Continuous Wear)	Gas Permeable
Vision	Good	Good	Good	Excellent (inc. astigmatism)
Comfort	Excellent	Good	Excellent	Good (after adaptation)
Convenience	Good	Average	Excellent	Good
Replacement	Daily–1 month	3–12 months	1 month	6–24 months
Solutions	No (daily) Yes (monthly)	Yes	No	Yes

Fitting of contact lenses and current legislation

Fitting contact lenses

The fitting of contact lenses and its management are strictly governed by the College of Optometrists and the various Optician Acts 1989. This is important to safeguard the public. Following the preliminary assessment of a prospective patient, the optometrist has a duty to ensure that each individual patient is fitted with the most appropriate lens type to give optimum vision for the required use. He or she has a duty to provide the patient with an appropriate lens care regimen and detailed written instructions on the use and wear of the lenses as well as the proposed aftercare schedule. When fitting each individual new contact lens wearer, the optometrist should ensure that:

a. The patient has had a recent eye examination

b. The type of lens and lens care regime are suitable and appropriate for the patient.

c. Prior to the fitting, the patient receives information and has a reasonable understanding of:

- the specific advantages and disadvantages of the lens types suitable for the patient.

- the care systems required by the different lens types and the total estimated costs.

d. Following the fitting, the patient is provided with full written instructions on:

- the insertion and removal of lenses, their care, storage, disinfection and cleaning

- the wearing schedule for the lenses

- the initial programme of aftercare and the need for regular scheduled contact lens check-ups thereafter

- the importance of seeking professional advice immediately any problem or discomfort is experienced and how and where to obtain that advice both during and outside normal office hours

- the importance of seeking professional advice before changing to a solution which has not already been recommended as suitable by the practitioner.

e. Appropriate elements of the instructions are given in writing to comply with the Medical Devices Directive.

f. The patient is advised of any required changes in the type of lens, lens wearing pattern or recommended hygiene regimen. Such advice should be given to the patient in writing and recorded clearly in the patient's records.

g. The same degree of care is required when fitting a patient with plano contact lenses as when fitting a patient with powered contact lenses. This includes adequate instruction on solutions, hygiene and handling. This is particularly important if the lenses are simply seen by the patient as 'fashion accessories' as this belief may lead to a more haphazard care regime. Patients should be advised strongly that they should not share their lenses as to do so carries a serious health risk.

Taken from http://www.college-optometrist.org (accessed 3 February 2006).

If the optometrist delegates any part of the patient's care to an un-qualified colleague the optometrist retains full responsibility for this.

Advice notes for patients are a useful aid to encouraging patient compliance. An effective recall system is important to encourage patients' regular attendance for scheduled contact lens check-ups. Where the optometrist refers the patient to be fitted by an appropriately qualified registered dispensing optician, the patient should still receive a full eye examination at appropriate intervals as determined by the clinical judgement of the prescribing optometrist.

The Optician's Act 1989 s25 (1A) states that 'a registered optometrist must not fit a contact lens for an individual unless:

a. Where the duty to give an individual a signed written prescription under section 26(2) below arises, he has the particulars of such a prescription given to the individual within the period of two years ending on the date the fitting begins and

b. The fitting begins before any re-examination date specified in that prescription'.

Therefore, if the patient is overdue for an eye examination, i.e. they have not had their eyes examined for more than 2 years, it is illegal for the optometrist to fit the patient with contact lenses (without examining the patient first so that they can issue a new prescription).

The Optician's Act defines fitting of a contact lens as:

a. Assessing whether a contact lens meets the needs of the individual and, where appropriate,

b. Providing the individual with one or more contact lenses for the use during a trial period.

THINKING POINT

TAKE A FEW MINUTES TO REFLECT ON THIS SCENARIO.
(Please note that this can be a typical presentation in the ophthalmic accident and emergency department.)

Mary Cheong is a 19-year-old law student who has been wearing soft gas permeable contact lenses for the past seven months. She rents a room in London and works all weekend to make ends meet. She lives among college friends in a crowded flat. Mary does not eat healthily. She has developed an acute red, painful eye for the past 2 days and her left vision is very blurred and sensitive to light. On assessment it became evident to the health practitioner that Mary was not complying with her contact lens care and hygiene regimen.

Discuss how the health practitioner would assess Mary on arrival at the Accident and Emergency department.

What specific information would the health practitioner be seeking to indicate that Mary was non-compliant?

What supporting evidence would Mary require to promote a positive attitude toward contact lens care?

Conclusion

This chapter has discussed one of the significant current issues and future challenges for ophthalmic practitioners, namely, the importance of good hygiene and effective contact lens care. It is essential that practitioners follow correct procedures for cleaning and disinfecting lenses, implements, instruments and surfaces in the contact lens room. Their contribution will help significantly to reduce the incidence of infection.

Education of the contact lens wearer remains the key future challenge in trying to prevent lens-related complications, especially as the number of contact lens wearers has steadily increased over the past decade. Contact lenses are medical devices and therefore patient screening and ongoing monitoring are essential to ensure their proper use.

References

Bacon, A.S., Fraser, D.G., Dart, J.K.G., Matheson, M., Ficker, L.A., and Wright, P. (1993). 'A review of seventy two consecutive cases of Acanthamoeba Keratitis 1984-1992.' *Eye* 7: 719–25.

British Contact Lens Association (BCLA). 'Lens wearing schedules and the need for cleaning.' http:www.bcla.org.uk/wearing_schedules.asp (last accessed on 13 February 2006).

Dart, J. (1993). 'The epidemiology of contact lens related disease in the United Kingdom.' *Contact Lens Ophthalmology* 19 (4): 241–5.

Dart, J. (1995). 'Clinical features of Acanthamoeba keratitis.' *Commumity Health Eye Journal* 8 (15): 1–3.

Ferriman, A. (1991). 'Risk to sight from 24 hour contact lens, say doctors.' *Observer Newspaper* 26 May 1991.

Miller, M.J., and Ahearn, D.G. (1987). 'Adherence of Pseudomonas aeruginosa to hydrophilic contact lenses and other substrata.' *Journal of Clinical Microbiology* 25: 1392–7.

Moore, M. (1990). 'Acanthamoeba keratitis and contact lens wear: the patient is at fault.' *Cornea* 9 (Supplement): 33–5.

Mowrey-Mckee, M.F., Monnat, K., and Sampson, H.J. (1992). 'Microbial contamination of hydrophilic contact lenses. Part 1: Quantitation of microbes on patient worn and handled lenses.' *Contact Lens Association of Ophthalmologists Journal* 18: 87–91.

Optician's Act (1989) S.25 (1A) http://www.college.optometrists.org (last accessed on 3 February 2006).

Polse, K.A. (1991). 'Contact lens research – a model for the 1990s.' *Journal of American Optometric Association* 62 (3): 162–4.

Rakow, P.L. (1993). 'Managing contact lens non-compliance.' *Journal of Ophthalmic Nursing and Technology* 12 (1): 47–8.

Rakow, P.L. (1999). 'Hypoxia and contact lens wear.' *Journal of Ophthalmic Nursing and Technology* 18 (1): 29–33.

Reichert, R., and Stern, G.A. (1984). 'Quantitation of adherence of bacteria to human corneal epithelial cells.' *Archive Ophthalmology* 102: 1394–5.

Schein, O.D., Glynn, R.J., Poggio, E.C., Seddon, J.M., and Kenyon, K.P. (1989). 'The relative risk of ulcerative keratitis among users of daily wear contact lenses.' *New England Journal of Medicine* 321: 773–8.

Seal, D.V., and Kirkness, C.M. (1995). 'Acanthamoeba keratitis and contact lens wear: the need for a global strategy for prevention of corneal infection.' *Community Eye Health* 8 (15): 4–6.

Stern, G.A. (1990). 'Pseudomonas keratitis and contact lens wear. The eye/lens is at fault.' *Cornea* 9 (Supplement): 536–8.

Stern, G.A. (1998). 'Contact lens associated bacterial keratitis: Past, present and future.' *The Contact Lens Association of Ophthalmologists Journal* 24: 52–6.

Chapter 5

Managing common eye disorders in the outpatient department

Ramesh Seewoodhary

Common eye disorders
Visual acuity assessment

Introduction

Chapter 4 provided an overview of the uses and complications of contact lenses, and it was evident that the magnitude of these eye complications ranged from minor to severely sight-threatening. Chapter 4 also addressed the issue of patient compliance and adopting a healthy regime. Many patients are advised to wear refractive contact lenses for conditions such as myopia, or as therapeutic contact lenses for disorders such as severe dry eyes, and keratoconus. Such conditions are often followed up in the ophthalmic outpatient department for monitoring and evaluation.

Chapter 5 therefore discusses the management of patients presenting with common eye disorders in the outpatient department. The reader needs to be aware that many patients who attend the outpatient department clinic may be contact lens wearers and it is the duty of all healthcare practitioners to give accurate and appropriate advice. Particular attention needs to be paid to underlying disorders such as conjunctivitis, blepharitis, styes, chalazion, and dry eyes.

All patients will require a thorough visual assessment and this means that the healthcare practitioner must have a working knowledge of these common presentations (Marsden, 2006). For medico-legal reasons, all ophthalmic patients require visual acuity assessment and this must be documented correctly on the patient's case notes (Seewoodhary 1983). Some patients may present with a refractive disorder in which case the patient should be referred to the optician for corrective lenses. Driving with blurred vision is very dangerous (Holden and Resnikoff, 2002). Visually disabling refractive error affects a significant proportion of the world population, occurs in both genders, in all age groups, and in all ethnic groups. It is also the easiest to cure (Holden and Resnikoff, 2002).

The current challenging issues highlighted in this chapter include (1) decision-making as to whether to continue follow-up patient care, (2) recognition of complications, (3) patient compliance, (4) omission of visual acuity recording. The significance of these issues becomes important when the patient develops ocular complications, or the patient seeks compensation as a result of visual loss.

According to a detailed survey of drivers' vision on road safety in 1997 by the Automobile Association, one out of every two motorists have been found to have defective vision in one eye (AA, 1995). This clearly indicates a worrying trend for all of us who are road users. Thus, regular eye testing is essential.

Common eye disorders

Common eye disorders

Common eye disorders form the majority of eye problems encountered in the ophthalmic outpatient department (Foster, 2005). Some of the more commonly seen eye complaints are shown in Table 5.1. It is important to emphasise that Table 5.1 is merely a guide to signs and symptoms of the more common eye disorders.

Table 5.1

Common eye complaints and possible signs and symptoms

Condition	Patient may complain of	You might observe
Conjunctivitis	Sore eye; gritty sensation in the eye; tearing; eyelids sticking together in the morning	Inflammation; tearing; discharge
Cataract	Misty, cloudy, or blurred vision; problems with glare in bright light	Milky white looking pupil (not always obvious in the early stages)

Glaucoma	Pain in the eyeball (ache); blurred vision; headache (often asymptomatic until quite late in the course)	Differences in when you and the patient can first see 'hands' in a 'confrontation' test
Foreign body	Pain in the eye; gritty sensation	Inflammation of the eye; tearing
Stye (hordeolum)	Pain in the eyelid	Localised eyelash follicle inflammation; yellow-headed swelling on the eyelid
Shortsight (myopia)	Being unable to see clearly in the distance	Patient squinting to see in the distance; decreased distance acuity on testing
Longsight (hypermetropia)	Being unable to read small print	Patient having obvious difficulty reading; decreased near acuity on testing
Macular degeneration	A gradual deterioration in central vision; straight lines appearing curved	Patient having difficulty in seeing directly in front
Dry eyes	Persistent, dry, gritty sensation in the eye; diminished vision	Inflammation; mucous discharge

A thorough inspection of the outside of the eye should include checking for any skin lesions or growths and inflammatory signs such as swelling, redness, warmth and/or tenderness. Abnormalities may occasionally be obvious, e.g. discharge or drooping of one or both eyelids (ptosis), asymmetry, and motor problems with the lids or protrusion (proptosis). However, even in the absence of obvious problems, all complaints of eye trouble should be treated seriously and specialists consulted where necessary. The pathologies underlying ocular symptoms are manifold and may reflect localised or systemic disorder.

Blepharitis

Blepharitis is the commonest lid problem encountered (Seewoodhary, 1983). The lid margins are red and thickened and show crust formation or squamous debris. Meibomian orifices are often blocked and meibomian glands inflamed. *Staphylococci aureus* or *epidermidis* may play a role in its production and may contribute to the associated conjunctivitis and punctuate keratitis.

Management involves twice daily lid hygiene. The lid margins are cleaned carefully with sodium bicarbonate lotion. Antibiotic ointment is usually prescribed for the lid margins. Warm compress with a moistened flannel increased the fluidity of the tarsal gland oils. Patient compliance is essential to prevent recurrence.

Stye

Styes are most common in young children and may occur singly or in crops affecting one or both lids. A stye is an acute infection of the lash follicle commonly caused by *Staphylococcus aureus*. It starts as a localised micro-abscess characterised by a tender, red, expanded lesion at the lid margin. The diagnosis is made by confirming the proximity of the stye to the lash base (Wybar and Kerr-Muir 1984).

It has been established that the Staphylococcal reservoir is located in the base of the follicle. A high percentage of the population are carriers of *Staphylococcus aureus* and are usually asymptomatic. The reason why some individuals develop styes and others do not is not known.

Styes respond favourably to hot bathing and topical antibiotic. When a crop of styes has subsided it is important to maintain lid hygiene to diminish factors such as marginal blepharitis which may encourage further episode of infection. Most severe styes are more common in diabetes. It may be necessary to prescribe a course of systemic antibiotic in resistant cases.

Chalazion

A chalazion is a granuloma within a tarsal oil gland or set of glands. Like the stye, there is an association with marginal blepharitis and particularly with meibomianitis (Vaughan and Asbury 2008). There is always abnormality of the meibomian orifices related directly to the chalazion. A chalazion may be sited anywhere along the lid. If a chalazion is on the lid margin it may be difficult to distinguish from a stye. However, a stye is always centred around a lash, while a marginal chalazion expands the posterior of the lid margin which contains the meibomian orifices.

When acutely inflamed there is accompanying infection with cellulitis and possibly abscess formation. There is a tender swelling within the substance of the lid with a variable degree of overlying redness. An acute chalazion may point and discharge inwards through the tarsal plate when it will be accompanied by conjunctivitis and discharge. More rarely the abscess points outwards through the tarsal plate, producing a collar stud lesion which may further discharge anteriorly through the lid skin.

The majority of chalazae develop as chronic granulomata which are relatively painless and merely produce a persistent lid swelling which can lead to visual disturbance by an effect on corneal shape. The overlying skin is not red but on eversion of the lid a localised redness and swelling of the torsal conjunctiva may be seen.

In the acute stage the patient is advised to use hot compress and a course of systemic antibiotic may be prescribed for five days. Lid hygiene is important as sometimes the lid margins may be red and crusty. A non-infected chalazion is managed surgically by incision and curettage under local anaesthesia. Successful curettage removes the necrotic centre of the chalazion. Firm padding over the initial three or four hours minimises the amount of blood which fills this space. Antibiotic ointment is applied daily for two days to prevent secondary infection. The patient should be informed and reassured that the swelling will not subside immediately but may take some weeks to do so.

A suspected lesion must be biopsied as very rarely a meibomian gland carcinoma may mimic a chalazion. All patients with symptomatic chalazae should be referred for ophthalmic assessment. Suspicion should be highest in the case of recurrent chalazion, recurring at the site of previous incision curettage.

Myopia and Hypermetropia

Myopia (short sight) is a condition in which there is a problem with distance vision, i.e. objects viewed from a distance appear out of focus. It usually occurs because the eyeball is 'too long', resulting in the image being optimally focused in front of the retina. However, in the special case of presbyopia, difficulty with distance vision may be related primarily to a diminished ability to accommodate. Myopia can be corrected by the use of appropriate strength concave lenses, (Seewoodhary, 2001).

An individual with hypermetropia (long sight) will not necessarily have any significant problem with either distance or near vision. Accommodation may be able to compensate for the eyeball being 'too short'. However, with increasing age, hypermetropic individuals may experience problems with their near vision and often their distance vision as well. In hypermetropia, the image is focused at a point beyond the retina. The condition can be corrected by the use of appropriate strength convex lenses.

Holden and Resnikoff (2002) discuss optometry as part of the eye care team. They highlight the need for glasses and stress the importance of this as a public eye health opportunity not to be missed. Refractive care provides excellent access to the population for screening of more serious eye problems such as cataract and diabetes. Sight testing programmes in all schools are an important element of eye care. It should not be necessary for any child to struggle in school, to learn with uncorrected refractive error. Nor should any older person be called upon to spend thirty to forty years without glasses, to see to read or sew or to manage a job. Optometrists thus play a key role in improving people's vision. Good eye sight is a precious gift.

Dry eye

Tears are a complex secretion derived from the lacrimal gland, the tarsal glands and the conjunctival goblet cells. Their role is to lubricate the conjunctival and corneal epithelial cells as well as preventing infection. This is because they carry protective antibodies and antibacterial agents such as lysozyme. A good tear film provides a smooth optical refracting surface to the eye and prevents corneal dryness (Vaughan and Asbury, 2008).

This film is in three layers:

a. an outermost lipid layer secreted by the tarsal glands

b. a middle watery layer from the lacrimal and accessory lacrimal glands

c. an innermost mucin layer derived from the conjunctiva, covering the corneal microvilli.

Dry eye is a frequent condition, and though serious complications are rare, the discomfort suffered by a patient can be considerable. In dry eyes, there can be an error of quantity or quality of the tears and also of the tear film. One of the three components of the tear film can become deficient. A lack of mucin leads to poor lubrication of the corneal epithelium and subsequent irritation. Mucin deficiency is found in trachoma, ocular pemphigoid and avitaminosis A. Lipid deficiencies occur in chronic blepharitis or in post-radiation damage where secreting cells are scarred. Insufficient lipid causes rapid evaporation of the watery layer. Deficiency of the aqueous layer occurs in lacrimal gland excision or in kerato-conjunctivitis sicca, where the lacrimal gland secreting cells become incapable of producing secretions or scarred ducts prevent egress of tears.

The symptoms of dry eyes include burning, itching, or gritty eyes. The patient will experience the symptoms frequently in dry, warm environments where tear evaporation is highest. Irritants in the atmosphere such as tobacco smoke will serve to exacerbate the symptoms. Situations in which the blink rate is reduced, e.g. prolonged reading will make matters worse.

Dry eye patients are always at risk of infection from bacteria, viruses and fungi. Patients presenting with a history of recurrent eye infection should be considered as a suspect dry eye case. The patient may complain of mucous strands lying in the conjunctival sac. These strands are attached to the corneal epithelium and may strip off some of this layer to cause corneal abrasion. The symptoms become acute with the patient seeking emergency help. Blurred vision is associated with dry eyes as the optical tear film becomes altered.

There are several simple tests which will aid in the diagnosis of dry eye:

1. Tear break up time of less than 10 seconds. This is assessed using a slit lamp bio-microscope. Rapid tear break up time leads to an increased frequency of blinking.

2. Schirmer's tear test measurement of less than 10mm in 5 minutes is considered positive. This test is not always reliable because reflex tearing can occur when the strips are inserted in the conjunctiva sac.

3. Rose Bengal dye staining of the phospholipids layer of the dead cells of the conjunctiva and cornea is a reliable test to diagnose dry eyes.

4. Slit lamp examination of the outer anterior segment will reveal lack of tear meniscus on the lid margin as well as the

state of the tear film when stained with fluorescein or when dry cells are stained with Rose Bengal.

5. Patient history often gives useful clues of the causes of dry eyes. For example, symptoms are classical, drug history may reveal the patient is on antidepressants, diuretics, antihistamine, beta blockers, atropine drops, nasal decongestants, etc.

The medical history is very helpful as dry eyes are often associated with thyrotoxicosis, rheumatoid arthritis, lack of vitamin A etc. There is no cure but the aim of the treatment is to relieve the patient's discomfort and to reduce the risk of serious complications such as infections. Treatment consists of either conserving those tears being formed or adding to them artificial tears. Conserving tears can be achieved by punctual occlusion by gelatine plug which is temporary or by punctual cauterisation which is permanent. Tears replacement therapy is by using artificial tears such as Lacri-lube, hypromellose. Mucolytic agents may be of value in breaking up the tenacious mucous filaments. Susceptible patients must keep away from smoky rooms, warm, dry atmospheres and poorly ventilated rooms.

Contact lens wear is usually contra-indicated in severe dry eyes as the cornea may become prone to ulceration and scarring. Any allergic reaction to preservatives must be taken note of and avoided. Sno tears have a long track record and are not liable to cause hypersensitivity reactions. Sno tears contain a wetting agent (polyvinyl alcohol 1.4% w/v) which will act as a stabiliser for the tear film, thereby increasing the tear break up time. Reducing the rate of tear evaporation and minimising development of dry spots. Any underlying causes must be attended to, e.g. vitamin A supplements, or treatment of thyroid eye disease etc. The wearing of goggles can provide a very local high humidity environment, thus reducing the loss of fluid through evaporation.

In all cases however, the aim of treatment should be:

a. lessening of patient's symptoms

b. lengthening of tear break up time

c. reduction in the areas of Rose Bengal staining (the dry spots)

d. avoidance of serious complications such as permanently damaged cornea and loss of visual acuity resulting from infections.

Should infection occur, then this should be adequately treated with antibiotics topically.

Dry eyes are troublesome eyes with potential to blindness. The earlier it is diagnosed and managed the less the chance of serious problems.

Visual acuity assessment

Visual acuity assessment

The issue of driving with eye problems concerns all of us. The DVLA (1999) is totally responsible for deciding whether an individual is permitted to drive. It demands that all drivers inform them of any existing eye condition or illness that may impair their driving ability. While doctors may be required to provide medical reports for the DVLA, they are not expected to stop their patients from driving (Keightley 1997). Ophthalmic practitioners have a duty to advise patients if they fail to meet legal driving requirements and inform them of their legal position.

Testing distance & near vision

Assessment of visual function is most commonly carried out through estimation of visual acuity (the 'sharpness' of definition with which an object or letter can be seen). Distance vision and near (or reading) visual acuity is usually estimated by testing. Each eye is tested separately.

For distance vision, a Snellen's chart is used (Figure 5.1, page 114). With one eye covered at a time the patient is asked to view the chart from a distance of 6m and to read down to the smallest letter that he or she can see. Distance or 'outdoor' spectacles should be worn if used.

Visual acuity is measured to assess central and peripheral vision. It is recorded to aid diagnosis, to monitor the progress of eye disorders and for insurance purposes (i.e. compensation claims after an eye injury (Seewoodhary, 1983).

Recording distance visual acuity

Sit the patient 6 metres from the Snellen's chart (Figure 5.1). Occlude one eye and ask the patient to read as much as possible of the chart with the other eye, starting from the top. Normal vision is 6/6: the numerator represents the distance from the chart and the denominator represents the row of letters read. Each letter subtends an angle of 5 minutes of arc at the nodal point of the eye. If the patient reads the top letter only at 6 metres from the chart, this is recorded as 6/60. The practitioner should record on the notes whether the eye is being tested with spectacles, contact lenses or unaided.

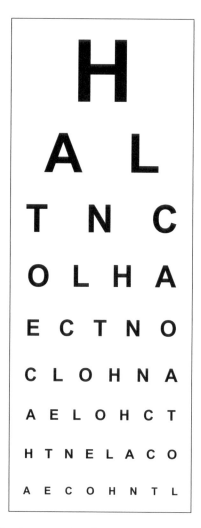

Figure 5.1

Snellen's chart is the standard equipment for measuring distance visual acuity. (Seewoodhary, 1983)

If a patient cannot read to 6/6, a pin-hole disc is used to test for central vision; this also helps to correct refractive error in an ametrophic eye (e.g. myopia). If the patient fails to read the top letter he is moved closer to the chart, 1 metre at a time, until the top letter is read (e.g. 2/60). A pin-hole disc is then used at 6 metres only.

If the patient fails to read at 1 metre, he or she is asked to count fingers at a normal distance of 0.3 metres; this is entered as 'counting fingers' in the notes. If the patient cannot count fingers, he is asked if he can see hand movements, and this is entered as 'hand movements' in the notes. Failing that, a torch is shone at the four quadrants of the eye to see if the patient can perceive light. This is entered as 'light perception' and the quadrant noted. If the patient fails to perceive light, this is simply entered as 'no perception of light'.

Near visual acuity assessment

Near vision, or reading vision, is usually tested by means of a reading card. This card usually has passages of text printed on it and, like Snellen's chart it consists of black letters on a white background. The patient is asked to hold the card at 33cm and to read the smallest print that he/she can easily read. When administering this test, it should be borne in mind that some individuals may be unable to carry out the test satisfactorily for reasons that are unrelated to their acuity, e.g. they may have difficulty in reading. These tests, which health practitioners will find relatively easy to administer, can indicate the need for spectacles or simply a new prescription to correct some problems of long and short sight.

Jaeger's types represent a random series of different sizes of printer's type, the smallest being J1 and the largest J20, but the modern N types are more exact because they are based on the point measurement of the height of a body of letters used in printing (one point = 1/72 inch). The letters are of ten different sizes – N5 (which equals five points), N6, N8, N10, N12, N14, N18, N24, N36, N60. A modification of the Sheridan-Gardiner test using 'reduced' Snellen types may be used for assessing the near vision in the young (Wybar and Kerr-Muir, 1984). A near visual acuity of N5 is equivalent to 6/12.

Testing peripheral vision

Typically, when we look straight ahead at an object, we are aware of being able to see other objects in our environment, even though we are not looking directly at them. These objects fall within our visual field and represent our peripheral or side vision. In conditions such as glaucoma, some people can suffer a progressive and insidious loss of peripheral vision, leaving them with sometimes considerable problems due to having to manage with tunnel-like vision. If the condition remains untreated it can result in blindness.

Health practitioners can estimate the extent of a patient's visual field by carrying out a simple confrontation test. In this test, the practitioner sits directly opposite the patient and a few feet away. The patient is then instructed to cover his or her left eye while the right eye is directed to the practitioner's left eye. The practitioner then asks the patient to maintain his or her gaze and identify the number of fingers shown by the nurse who holds his or her hand in different areas of the patient's peripheral vision, e.g. upper left, lower left, upper right and lower right. The practitioner can see whether the patient maintains his or her gaze, as he or she is in eye to eye contact. If the nurse's fingers that are shown are presented at about half way between the practitioner and patient, the respective visual fields should be approximately the same. This allows the practitioner to compare visual fields with the patient. Each eye should be tested separately.

THINKING POINT

TAKE A FEW MINUTES TO REFLECT ON YOUR MOST RECENT OPHTHALMIC EXPERIENCE IN YOUR PRACTICE AREA.

Consider a young patient or an elderly patient attending with an eye complaint of a longstanding nature. The patient may present to the ophthalmic department without a referral letter or have been referred by his or her primary care doctor.

Discuss with a colleague the following points of interest and say what you have learnt from this reflective exercise:

a. What pertinent questions would you ask when assessing the patient?

b. How would you assess the patient's visual acuity and how would you evaluate the findings of the visual acuity findings? Why is visual acuity recording important?

c. Explain how the history taking has enabled you to make a provisional diagnosis.

d. Discuss the significance of obtaining a medical history, drug history, and any other histories of relevance.

e. What are the main anxieties experienced by ophthalmic patients attending the outpatient department?

Conclusion

This chapter has explored some common ophthalmic disorders encountered in the eye clinic. The importance of patient assessment was also addressed with particular reference to the assessment of visual acuity and how to record it. Driving with good eye sight is the responsibility of all road users.

The eye conditions discussed related to non-emergency ophthalmic disorders. However, complexities do occur when each patient is assessed and cared for. The Thinking Point provides the reader with an ideal opportunity for reflection on the key issues addressed within the chapter. The main issues and challenges discussed in this chapter are also those faced by practitioners working in the ophthalmic Operating Theatre. As previously pointed out, non-emergency ophthalmic disorders can sometimes become complex after the patient's assessment and will require further surgical intervention as part of the ongoing treatment. Patient assessment and the accurate documentation of visual acuity assessment are equally important for the ophthalmic operating theatre practitioner prior to commencing any surgical procedure. These issues will be highlighted again in the next chapter.

References

Automobile Association (1995). 'Would you see this car coming?' *Road Safety* Summer 35. London: AA.

Driver and Vehicle Licensing Agency (1999). *At a Glance Guide to Current Medical Standards for Fitness to Drive*. Swansea: DVLA.

Foster, A. (2005). 'Red eye: the role of primary care.' *Community Eye Health Journal* 18 (53): 69.

Holden, B.A., and Resnikoff, M.D. (2002). 'The role of optometry in vision 2020.' *Community Eye Health Journal* 15 (43): 33–6.

Keightley, S.J. (1997). 'Visual standards in driving.' Royal College of Ophthalmologists. *Focus*. Summer. London: RCO.

Marsden, J. (2006). *Ophthalmic Care*. West Sussex: John Wiley and Sons Ltd.

Seewoodhary, M. (1983). 'Common presentations in accident and emergency.' *Nursing: the add-on Journal of Clinical Nursing* 2 (17): 498–500.

Seewoodhary, R. (2001). 'Degenerative myopia.' *Ophthalmic Nursing* 4 (4): 14–17.

Vaughan, D., and Asbury, T. (2008). *General Ophthalmology*, 17th edition. York: McGraw-Hill.

Wybar, K., and Kerr-Muir, M. (1984). *Ophthalmology*. London: Bailliere Tindall.

Chapter 6

Ophthalmic theatre practice

Lavona Dampies

Current issues for the ophthalmic theatre practitioner

Advancing ophthalmic theatre practice through nurse-led initiatives

Moving ophthalmic surgical services into the community

Future constraints in the operating theatre

Introduction

The preceding chapters look at the patient being correctly diagnosed and treated in the ophthalmic outpatient as well as the Accident and Emergency departments. Both are areas where the ophthalmic practitioner might have limited contact with the patient, but where effective history taking and a sound knowledge of eye disease is paramount for the diagnosis and treatment of patients when seen in these areas. Patients might also need to receive further treatment in the operating theatre after being examined in these departments. This would be the area where the preparation of patients requiring surgery would begin, as some medical conditions might have to be treated as emergencies.

This therefore highlights the need for the operating theatre practitioner to understand the procedures and tests carried out in these departments and how they aid the further treatment of patients in theatre. This chapter will explore some of the current and future challenges for the practitioner working within the ophthalmic theatre.

The role of the theatre practitioner has always seemed

ambiguous to the general public. Mardell (1998) highlights that doubts arise about the job of theatre nursing being nursing, with a high percentage of patients not realising that nurses work in the operating theatres. As the role of these practitioners was seen as technical, they were characterised as 'quick fit mechanics' for bodies (Mardell and Rees, 1998). This chapter will thus aim to critically explore and reflect on the current and future practices influencing ophthalmic theatre nursing. These practitioners face daily challenges of providing therapeutic, patient centred care against a growing, highly technical environment (Evans and Taylor, 2006). This clearly indicates that practitioners need to be highly skilled to cope with these demands. The Nursing and Midwifery Council (NMC, 2008) have clearly set out the account-abilities of practitioners when caring for patients, incorporating the identification and reduction of risk.

It is important not to forget the political, social and economic influences that may drive many of these changes, thus dictating the future of the theatre practitioner. This includes the knowledge and skills to link evidence to practice, resulting in the delivery of total quality patient care and choice. This emphasises the need for more efficient and effective ways of working, ultimately leading to performance improvement within set budgets and government targets. This includes the awareness of shortage of funds for training and specialist update, as well as the use of these funds to cover other budget shortfalls.

Current issues for the ophthalmic theatre practitioner

Managerial issues

Current issues

The environment in which we exist is continuously in flux. In the ever-changing NHS that constantly demands new services, products and ways of working, innovation is vital (Moroney and Knowles 2006). This involves staying up-to-date with procedural, social and political changes. Some of these rapid changes could also be linked to the demand of the high quality of care patients need to receive, set out as a ten-year plan of modernisation (DoH, 1998). Triggers for change can be positive or negative, resulting from managerial growth, a drive for continuous improvement, responses to new technology and/or a shift in the market (Westwood 2001).

The government has a big effect on the issues surrounding ophthalmic theatre practitioners. These are driven by White Papers on reforming the National Health Service (NHS), and specific national standards known as National Service Frameworks (NSFs). Linking the Action on Cataracts (DoH, 2000a) with the NSF for Older People (DoH, 2002) resulted in an improved quality of life for millions (DoH, 2001a, NICE, 2004), especially the elderly, by reducing falls and maintaining their independence. It is therefore clear that older people with visual problems are in need of significantly improved access to treatment centres providing cataract surgery.

Reform has been developed through the NHS Plan (1997, 2000b) (Montgomery, 2003), resulting in extensive change under the Health Act 1999, and the Health and Social Care Act 2001, especially related to the reduction in waiting list times. The impact was huge, as extra operations had to be done on existing lists, and some operating lists had to be done out of hours to accommodate these requirements. Theatre practitioners have been doing a great deal of 'extra' work to meet the requirements of the waiting list initiatives (Campbell, 2000). These extra lists are still being done on an 'ad hoc' basis to enable ophthalmic departments to stay within their required waiting times, leading to theatre practition-ers being tired and going off sick, which in turn causes stress on the rest of the team having to cope with the absence. This places additional stress on the Trust who then has to aggressively manage sickness absence in a drive to increase productivity. Patients may also suffer the cancellation of surgery due to these factors. A number of other demands and deficits remain unsolved, for example the longer wait for procedures that are not linked to tight waiting time controls before the implementation of the 18-week target. This government initiative requires that a patient wait no longer than 18 weeks for the start of their treatment, since referral from their GP.

The reduction of waiting times, the treatment of certain diseases, advancing medical and pharmaceutical technology, the need for constantly training practitioners, an ageing population, and the effect of the NHS plan all have financial implications for the operating theatre. Including the need for expensive or disposable consumables, higher patient and political expectations, this can in turn lead to overspends on budgets. Klein (2001) highlighted the poor economic status of the NHS during 1978/9 and 1989/90 when the overall budget ot the NHS was only increased by 1 per cent per year. We had to implement so many changes and keep up with the ever-changing technology, while still working within very tight budgets due to the slow increase of public funding of the service. However we have seen vast increases in finances during 1999–2005. This clearly highlights the complexity of economic pressures on healthcare policy and healthcare systems in all areas of the NHS. This situation is also not helped by the current financial climate we have within the NHS. Here leaders were in the past allowed to go over their yearly budget, by making adjustments for the following financial year and incorporating overspends within the new budgets. This is now a thing of the past as leaders are currently required to make a 2.5% saving on their budgets (Rogers and Taylor, 2007). The modern NHS now requires that the highest quality of care be provided at the lowest cost, through continuous service improvement. Payment by Results has also set the standard by which trusts are paid for work done on a case-by-case basis, and tariffs set on a national average hospital cost linked to more than 1,000 healthcare codes.

Patient expectation and choice is also having an impact on the theatre practitioner. This includes international efforts to strengthen the position of healthcare users within the healthcare system. Baggot (2004) highlights the declarations issued by the World Health Organisation (WHO) Regional Office for Europe (1994) and the Council of Europe (2000) stating the importance of patients' rights and patient participation in healthcare decision-making. This covers patient involvement/empowerment in a patient centred environment, where the patient makes the choice of the treatment they prefer, the time frame, as well as the centre where they would prefer to be treated. Increased patient choice could also have its own drawbacks. Some people may make more use of choice than others. Another problem is that if Foundation Trusts do not offer a specific service the Primary Care Trusts wants, then they can take business elsewhere. This could lead to a reduction in patient numbers, leading to a reduction in income and a diminished skill base that may lead to redundancies. But it could also be argued that specialist centres can lead to high standards of care, and an increased workload. The NHS may also suffer loss of income if they have increased competition from private providers of treatment having adverse affects on patient services. This was clearly experienced during the period of working to get the cataract waiting times within the expected government time frames.

The aforesaid formed the basis for 'patient-centred care' which placed emphasis on the role of the practitioner, highlighting the need to expand these roles, resulting in the formation of nurse-led services. The increased availability of healthcare information on the internet, television and media affects patient expectations of processes or services.

The above requires that a patient be fully informed about his or her condition and/or treatment to enable them to make any informed choice about their treatment and where they would like to obtain it. Here the importance of a well-informed theatre practitioner is emphasised again. The practitioner may be the person to support the patient or client with health guidance that has the person's needs as its focus, ensuring they do not influence the patient in the decision making, or coerce them into following instructions. This highlights a greater need for professional accountability, regulation and updated skills as patients are more enlightened about their care and health technology. By continuously updating their knowledge of evidence-based practice, practitioners can influence and increase the quality of care for patients and themselves. Such up-to-date knowledge is also of value, in the light of increasing rates of clinical negligence litigation. Here the National Institute of Clinical Excellence (NICE) and the NHS Institute for Innovation and Improvement (2005) rolled out a national improvement initiative on providing leadership development that results in clinical and cost effectiveness. The NHS Institute for Innovation and Improvement (DoH, 2001b) has also clearly highlighted the significance of clinical governance in managing patient care to ensure an optimum standard of care is delivered and maintained throughout the patient's stay in hospital.

Risk management cannot be removed from quality of care or clinical governance as it forms a link with both these subjects. NHS Trusts need to ensure that robust policies, procedures and protocols are in place to demonstrate to the Department of Health that they are compliant with clinical governance (Scott and Summerball, 2004). This is due to the fact that litigation costs the NHS around £1 billion a year and the fact that complications may lead to longer hospitalisation, healthcare-acquired infections and may result in the settlement of negligence claims. The NHS Litigation Authority (NHSLA, 2008) has put standards in place that they use to accredit Trusts against compliance. Risk management thus plays a crucial part of the operating practitioner's role, concentrating on the following areas:

- Reporting and investigating incidents and learning from them
- Ensuring that mistakes and errors are not repeated
- Ensuring that staff members are 'risk aware' and are active in managing risks.

This involves always aiming to achieve excellent results following any care rendered, and acting to identify and minimise risk to patients and clients, in accordance with the NMC (2008). This can be done by carrying out certain checks before the start of each operating list, or prior to the start of each operative procedure.

This is linked to clinical practice benchmarking and clinical governance, a process implemented by the government, whereby NHS organisations are accountable for continuous improvement of the quality of service rendered, maintaining high standards of care and creating an environment in which clinical excellence will flourish (DoH 1998, 2000b). Quality thus becomes the driving force of decision-making for the ophthalmic theatre practitioner, and at every level of the multi-disciplinary team, as stated by the Secretary of State for Health (1997, cited by Brocklehurst and Walshe, 1999). This includes national clinical standard setting, as well as robust and effective systems for assuring improved quality, with continuous auditing of services to ensure the quality challenge is met, through the identification of problems and resolving them as a learning curve without a blame culture.

The above also highlights further NICE Guidelines (2006) for vitreo-retinal (VR) surgery, including the use of disposable instruments not even available on the market, or the ones that are available not being suitable to use for the purpose it was designed for. This has a big financial implication, in a climate when staff members are urged to work within tight budget constraints.

Another guideline dictates that instruments should under no circumstances be moved from one instrument tray to another. In the incidence of defective instruments, the tray should then be removed from circulation until the repair or new instrument is received, with a further implication of having to keep all instruments and equipment used for a specific VR case together. This may require more instruments and equipment, e.g. Binocular Intra-ocular Microscopy (BIOM) systems, requiring more funds.

Difficulty in recruiting ophthalmic theatre practitioners can sometimes lead to staff shortages, and inappropriate skill mix (McColgan, 2006). One could argue that this problem may be linked to students not able to rotate through theatres during their training programme. This highlights the fact that some pre-registration education programmes still do not offer students experience in the operating department, which could be a limiting factor for recruitment and retention (Campbell, 2000). Another reason might be nurses not having an interest in the operating theatre as a workplace. Both could be due to a lack of knowledge about the role of a theatre practitioner, due to the fact that theatre practitioners used to work in isolation from the wards, and that theatre could have been seen as an institution on its own. By not investing time and money in the education of existing practition-ers, or by not committing to employ people without the appropriate theatre skills and investing in the training of these people, operating theatres may also be faced with staff shortages. The misunderstanding of Agenda for Change pay band assimila-tions could also have contributed to staff members resigning, rather than seeking clarification. In addition, some NHS Trusts embark on job cuts as a means of financial saving. This results in reduced staff numbers which leads to fewer placements for student nurses that might impact nursing in future.

Clinical issues

Treating the patient as a whole might not always be possible in the operating room, due to the limited time spent in that environment. It can thus be said that care is limited to the area in which the patient is treated. Patients may not understand why certain information is required by the theatre practitioner, and may also interpret such behaviour as intrusive and manipulative, while theatre practitioners may find it difficult to defend why they need to know specific details and to identify how the information would be used (Price, 2006). Yet it is imperative for the theatre practitioner to remember that they are treating a human being with attitudes, beliefs, morals, norms and feelings. Here mutual trust and respect is paramount, which has to be formed within a short time span.

When receiving a patient in theatre, it is the responsibility of the practitioner to follow the theatre check-in policy to ensure that the correct patient is checked in for the correct operative procedure. The Joint Commission on Accreditation of Healthcare Organisations (2004) now requires the surgeon to mark the operative site prior to the patient coming to theatre. Other checks should include the patient's full name, date of birth, operative site, and signed consent corresponding with the operative list, allergy status, and hospital number, both verbally and according to the patient's identity band (Scott and Summerball, 2004).

The increase in day surgery under local anaesthesia has meant a change in the role of the theatre practitioner, since they are more frequently close to patients who may be anxious and feeling vulnerable (Mardell 1998). Here privacy and dignity of the patient or client take precedence, by making the patient aware that he or she is 'in charge' of the situation surrounding the procedure, e.g. they may stop the operative procedure at any time during the intra-operative phase if the need arises to cough. The patient is thus empowered to be in control of their care, thus aiming to reduce the patient's anxiety in the operating theatre and achieve a speedy post-operative recovery. This clearly indicates that the ophthalmic theatre practitioner does not just pass the instruments to the surgeon during the surgery, or circulate for the scrub nurse, but has to assess the needs of the patient – highlighting the importance of the patient being aware of what is about to happen to him or her throughout the procedure, emphasising the need for accurate assessment of the patient's needs by an expert, ensuring their care is planned and rendered accordingly, resulting in effective communication between the multi-disciplinary team.

New methods of working are constantly taking shape. Here the new 'corneal inlay' procedure to correct myopia and reduce keratoconus is another example. This procedure involves the dissection of the peripheral layers of the cornea using suction via a machine, making two incisions into the cornea. A guide is introduced into the outermost layer where the inlay will be placed; the crescent shaped corneal ring is inserted to alter the shape of the cornea and reduce astigmatism. The cut is sealed with a single suture. The ophthalmic practitioner has to have a sound knowledge of their field, doing constant research on current practice, products and new techniques. This clearly highlights the need for access to training and/or funds for training. Here we should not forget the availability of funds to ensure departments are covered by bank or agency staff, to allow practitioners the necessary time to attend appropriate study sessions.

The role of a specialised ophthalmic theatre practitioner is highly skilled. It demands the ability to anticipate throughout the procedure and be ready to cope with any change or emergency when the need arises, without any surprises. Gone are the days of being the 'hand maiden' for the 'captain of the ship', and becoming 'lost behind a mask'. One of the hidden skills is that of non-verbal communication and being able to read each other's body language to enable support and rapid response in a crisis, acquired through experience. Changes in the role of the theatre practitioner resulted in the 'birth' of the peri-operative practitioner and peri-operative care. It thus includes the pre-, intra-, and post-operative phases of the patient's surgical experience. These changes, together with the rapidly changing technology, demand that the operating practitioner ensures that he or she stays up-to-date with these changes. Specialised professional knowledge is paramount whilst also being able to develop the ability to apply the knowledge, life skills and evidence-based research to practice. This requires the theatre practitioner to become more qualified, now gaining a degree, diploma or other relevant qualification (Rees, 1999).

Here an example is the way in which cataract surgery has progressed over the past ten years, from doing Extra-Capsular Cataract Extraction (ECCE) where the surgery was predominantly performed under general anaesthetic, and as an inpatient, to the Phaco-emulsification (Phaco) of the cataract (ultra-sonic emulsification of cataract under fluid irrigation and aspiration). Here a sound knowledge of both procedures was needed during the transition from one procedure to the other which had training implications for staff. Cataract surgery is now predominantly performed under local anaesthesia, done as a day case, and comparison studies have proved it to be an intrinsically safe procedure (Cooper, 1999). Cataract surgery is sophisticated, safe, quick and cost-effective (Batterbury and Bowling, 1999), which emphasises the fact that specialist ophthalmic practitioners are needed to assist during these procedures (as discussed in Chapter 1). The ophthalmic theatre practitioner is still required to have the ability to convert to ECCE and/or anterior vitrectomy if required when the posterior capsule is ruptured (Evans and Taylor, 2006).

As the aim of cataract extraction is to improve the vision of the patient, the theatre practitioner should have a sound knowledge of biometry and refractions to ensure the correct intra-ocular lens (IOL) is implanted into a patient. This involves a broad knowledge of the different types of IOLs available and their injectors where applicable, their A-constants, the size ranges, and ensuring the availability of the correct IOL. The ophthalmic theatre practitioner should understand the various features of the Phaco machine in use, being able to explain these to the surgeon when needed, and being able to troubleshoot should the need arise. Knowledge of the various machines is only one of the fundamentals the theatre practitioner should have. Here knowledge of the operative procedure, all equipment and instruments needed is also very important. The specialist training that this entails might cause pressure on the team, as staff members are required to leave the department during their training. By being very familiar with the anatomy, physiology and steps in the procedure, the practitioner can contribute to reducing the length of the surgical time, benefiting the patient's comfort and safety and reducing retinal toxicity from prolonged exposure to the microscope lights (Evans and Taylor, 2006).

The way in which the instruments are handed to the surgeon should allow them to continue operating during this stage without having to look away from the operating microscope and then losing their three-dimensional vision. The theatre practitioner should always adhere to safety measures when passing the instruments to prevent stab injuries. Instruments should thus be passed with the sharp ends downwards and placed firmly into the surgeon's hand, ready for use. A good practice is to confirm with the surgeon what you have placed in his or her hand, not forgetting the importance of knowing if the surgeon is right or left handed. This makes a real difference, as instruments do not need to pass from one hand to the other, reducing operative time and a reduced risk of injury in case an instrument is accidentally dropped during the extra manoeuvre.

Noise should be minimised as sudden patient or surgeon movement could have serious consequences for the surgical outcome (Evans and Taylor, 2006). Whispering should be avoided as it is a distraction to the surgeon working through a microscope. The patient should also be able to follow instructions from the surgeon. No telephones should be kept inside the operating theatre as they may cause a distraction if they ring during a surgical procedure. If there is a need to talk, do so at a stage during the surgical procedure when it would pose no risks to the surgery, and in a normal tone of voice.

Theatres should be specially laser proofed as stipulated by international guidelines, with theatre practitioners trained about the laser safety rules. Theatre practitioners should play an important part in ensuring the safe delivery of laser treatment to patient and staff. Staff should be aware of the following points:

- Protective eyewear should be used as lasers can cause irreversible damage to the eye. While treating the affected eye, a moist swab should cover the fellow eye of the patient receiving treatment.

- Practitioners should be aware that safety eyewear is not interchangeable between different laser machines, due to the difference in laser wavelength and power of machines.

- Reflections of laser beams are also damaging, so all surfaces near the operative field should be non-reflective. The laser is a fire hazard so regular maintenance is paramount.

- Laser safety signs should be in effect while the laser is in use. Practitioners should be aware of the emergency shut-off on the laser machine, as well as who the laser officer is in the event of any problems.

It is paramount for the ophthalmic theatre practitioner to be knowledgeable about the pharmacological agents and fluids used in the ophthalmic theatre during the delivery of patient care. This includes not using drug-containing preservatives within the eye as it may cause damage by toxicity. Drugs and fluids used within the eye should always be isotonic and preferably buffered (Evans and Taylor, 2006).

Control of infection forms an integral part of the role of the ophthalmic theatre practitioner. This includes infection risk to the patient as well as the theatre practitioner. Control of infection principles is governed by robust legislation, policies and procedures to reduce risks to both parties. They may be either non-clinical, relating to clothing, linen, clinical waste, or clinical, relating to policies of handwashing, practice, equipment, protective clothing (PPE) and the environment (McCulloch, 1998; Xavier, 1999). Infection control practice aims to:

- prevent the development of infection and
- prevent the transmission of existing infection.

Healthcare-associated infections (HCAIs) cost the NHS £1 billion a year, causing about 5,000 deaths, of which one-third could have been prevented (Chambers and Straub, 2006).

Acquiring a severe inflammation or infection of the eye during cataract or any other intra-ocular surgery can result in blindness. The operating theatre environment can pose a severe threat at any time, as research indicates that there are microscopic fibre particles in the air, which can enter the wound site during surgery (Pisani, 2004). Any loss of vision is a severe tragedy and will definitely affect the patient's quality of life. Management and preventative measures of minimising airborne fibre particles in the sterile ophthalmic theatre environment are thus paramount.

Evans and Taylor (2006) highlight that ophthalmic theatres should be designed to the same high specifications as other theatres. Specialised ventilation is required in the operating departments, ensuring the pressure inside the theatre is higher than that outside so that the air flows in one direction, away from the theatre with 20–30 air exchanges per hour. The ultimate goal is to contain, control and reduce hazards to patient and staff from airborne contaminants. NHS Estates (1998) states that clear management responsibility should be in place so that no doubt exists about who is responsible for the safe operation and maintenance of equipment. All practitioners must be educated on this issue, with the view of reducing ocular morbidity and cost to the NHS (Tingle, 2002). Practitioners should be aware that the lower limit of theatre temperature is 18 degrees Celsius before Health and Safety measures kick in. At present no upper limit is set, but an ideal temperature when operating on children should be about 25 degrees

Celsius (Clarke and Jones, 1998; cited by Evans and Taylor, 2006).

Endophthalmitis is a serious infection and is largely preventable by ensuring a clean and safe environment (DoH, 1998). All ophthalmic theatre personnel must have a working knowledge of microbiology, pathogens, theatre air filter systems, foreign fibres, and Trust policies to contribute towards patient safety and clinical governance principles. Levine and Snyder (1999) describe the commonest pathogens causing endophthalmitis as *Staphylococcus aureus*, which can be introduced at any time during the intra-operative phase. These are spherically shaped, arranged in clusters, and are aerobic gram-positive bacteria. Xavier (1999) highlights the fact that some patients are more vulnerable to infection, due to complex immunology and the individual's response to invading organisms. The source of infection is often unclear, ranging from surgical instruments, airborne particles, contaminated solutions, to patients' own microbiota. The infected eye becomes watery, red, and painful with photophobia, leading to decrease in vision. This may require emergency management to save sight (Levine and Snyder, 1999). Any delay or misdiagnosis can result in a poor outcome and vision loss.

The Department of Health has launched a new control of infection initiative, the 'Saving Lives' campaign. This is one of the national initiatives that should be followed by every hospital, emphasising that hospital staff should conform to the yearly control of infection update, with a website started to assist staff in this respect. This was then followed by 'The cleanyourhand campaign' where staff ensure that they protect their patients from the risk of infection, by cleaning their hands before and after every patient at the point where care is delivered. This campaign also acknowledges that visitors bring infection into the hospital, and encourages them to use alcohol gel as they enter the hospital, relying on the compliance of patients and visitors to use the prescribed alcohol hands rub to ensure we move towards combating hospital infections. Patients are also empowered to ask healthcare workers if their hands are clean.

This has further rolled out to the 'Bare arm policy'. Here everybody in direct patient care is not permitted to wear long sleeved clothes, wrist watches, or any device around their arms during care delivery. One plain metal band (wedding band) is permitted. This is due to the fact that jewellery may harbour bacteria and hinder the hand washing process.

Creutzfeldt-Jakob Disease (CJD) is a term that includes several similar brain diseases (NICE, 2004). Variant CJD (vCJD) is a similar condition, which was discovered in 1996, and is believed to be a human form of bovine spongiform encephalopathy (BSE) also known as 'mad-cow disease'. It is believed that CJD and vCJD are transmitted by prions, though this is still not completely certain. Prions are molecules of protein and unlike other germs (like bacteria and viruses) they cannot be easily disabled or killed with disinfectants or by heating. These patients have high concentrations of prions in particular tissues in their body, including the eye. This could thus lead to the possibility of transmitting of the disease to other patients. Although instruments have been decontaminated and sterilised after use on an infected patient, prion proteins may not be effectively destroyed by this process.

THINKING POINT

- Does your department have a policy for the handling of instruments used on a patient suspected of having CJD?
- Do you know the contents of this policy?
- Who would be the facilitator of this policy, in the absence of your leader?
- Do you understand the necessity to carry out the final procedure of this policy?

Advancing ophthalmic theatre practice through nurse-led initiatives

Advancing theatre practice

The European directive on reducing doctors' working hours, closely linked to another governmental enterprise of quality improvement, resulted in establishing the advancing the role of the nurse. Here the term 'Advanced Practice' suggests a level of practice that is beyond the requirement for initial registration with the NMC (Wilson and Bunnell, 2007). One of the problems experienced in ophthalmic practice was patients' surgery cancelled because they were unfit. Dealing with this problem led eventually to the introduction of the nurse practitioner role (Reveley et al., 2002).

This role started with the nurse being able to complete a pre-operative assessment, previously carried out by the doctor, if it was done at all (Wadsworth *et al.*, 2002). The nurse practitioner role soon expanded to include running minor operation lists and administering local anaesthesia prior to ocular surgery. The training for this role is normally done at local level. It includes training as a specialist ophthalmic theatre nurse, incorporating pre-op assessment. This suggests that the skills that the nurse possesses may be closely linked to those of a medic, but practitioners need to be aware of using these skills according to their clinical judgement as they will practice as autonomous practitioners. The Royal College of Nursing (RCN, 2005) highlighted that it is clear that these nurses are at the leading edge of transforming how health service are delivered, depending on their nursing skills, knowledge and experience. The RCN believes that growing and nurturing these roles is therefore critical to the development of patient-centred health services across the UK.

Moving surgical services into the community

Moving surgical services

This initiative helps to free some operating time for more specialised care in the bigger hospitals that could allow centres of excellence to flourish, while the patient would still receive the same quality specialist care if the more suitable day-case procedure is mobilised in these areas. It may also resolve some transport problems for the elderly patient group if they are treated closer to their home, causing less stress to the patient and leading to a reduction in transport costs.

Future constraints

Future constraints

Future constraints on the ophthalmic theatre practitioners are driven by the UK20/20 Vision Strategy which was launched to 'address inequalities' which lead to unnecessary blindness. This is partly linked to ophthalmic diseases caused through age, but this initiative will also aim to tackle avoidable blindness caused by glaucoma, cataract and age-related macular degeneration (AMD) (Royal College of Ophthalmologists, 2008). This initiative is closely linked to that of the World Health Organisation's Vision20/20 (WHO 2005). It has also become apparent that the need for treatment of patients with AMD will increase due to our aging population, and the new NICE guideline for treatment due to be initiated in August 2008. Many ophthalmic theatres do not have to worry about this practice, but we need to be mindful of hospitals that do not have the necessary sterile room facility in order to treat these patients in a clinic setting.

Conclusion

This chapter has attempted to explore some of the current and future challenges faced by the ophthalmic theatre practitioner, highlighting the highly technical environment ophthalmic theatre practitioners work in. This highly skilled and ever-changing environment requires the ophthalmic theatre practitioner to stay up-to-date with research, professional and clinical knowledge and skills. Practitioners also need to be aware of internal and external influences affecting their practice, and how to cope with or overcome them. They should also understand and embrace the principles of productivity improvement and efficiency of finances.

In order to improve patient care, the ophthalmic theatre practitioner needs to be aware of the role of the advanced practitioner, and the advantages of referring some of the practices into the community. Becoming an advanced practitioner, however, also requires a knowledge and understanding of the legal and ethical issues surrounding this role and the need to acknowledge the importance of professional accountability in an increasingly litigious society. Such issues form the basis for an in-depth discussion in the following chapter.

References

Baggot, R. (2004). *Health and Health Care in Britain*. 3rd Edition. Basingstoke, Hampshire: Palgrave Macmillan.

Batterbury, M., and Bowling, B. (1999). *Ophthalmology. An Illustrated Colour Text*. London: Churchill Livingstone.

Brocklehurst, N., and Walshe, K. (1999). 'Quality and the new NHS.' *Nursing Standard* 8 (13): 46–53.

Campbell, L. (2000). 'Waiting in the wings.' *British Journal of Perioperative Nursing* 10 (2): 298.

Chambers, C., and Straub, M. (2006). 'Standard principles for preventing and controlling infection. *Nursing Standard.* 20, 23, 57-65.

Clarke, P., and Jones, J. (eds) (1998). *Brigden's Operating Department Practice.* Edinburgh: Churchill Livingstone.

Cooper, J. (1999). 'Teaching patients in post-operative eye care: the demands of day surgery.' *Nursing Standard* 18 (13): 42–6.

Council of Europe (2000). *Recommendation No.R (2000) 5 of the Committee of Ministers to member states on the development of structures for citizen and patient participation in the decision-making process affecting health care.* Available on-line from: https://wcd.coe.int/ViewDoc.jsp?Ref = Rec(2000)5& Language = lanEnglish&Ver = original&Site = COE&BackColorInternet = DBDCF2 &BackColorIntranet = FDC864&BackColorLogged = FDC864 (Accessed June 2007).

Department of Health (1997). *The New NHS: Modern and Dependable.* London: HMSO.

Department of Health (1998). *A First Class Service: Quality in the New NHS.* London: HMSO.

Department of Health (2000a). *Action on Cataracts. Good Practice Guidance.* London: HMSO.

Department of Health (2000b). *The NHS Plan: A Plan for Investment: A Plan for Reform.* London: HMSO.

Department of Health (2001a). *National Service Framework for Older People.* London: HMSO.

Department of Health (2001b). *Good Practice in Consent Implementation Guide.* London: HMSO.

Department of Health (2002). *National Service Framework (NSF) for Older People: Meeting the Milestone (supporting documentation for NSF champions).* London: HMSO.

Evans, P., and Taylor, G. (2006). 'Ophthalmic theatre nursing.' In Marsden, J. (ed.) *Ophthalmic Care.* England: Wiley-Blackwell, pp. 183–208.

Joint Commission on Accreditation of Healthcare Organisations (2004). *Patient Safety Goals.* Online available from: http://www.jointcommission.org/Patient SafetyNationalPatientSafetyGoals/04_npsgs.htm. Accessed 1 April 2007.

Klein, R. (2001). *The New Politics of the NHS.* 4th Edition. Harlow, England: Pearson Prentice Hall.

Levine, J., and Snyder, R.W. (1999). 'Practical ophthalmic microbiology.' *Journal of Ophthalmic Nursing and Technology.* 18, 2.

Mardell, A. (1998). 'How theatre nurses perceive their role: a study.' *Nursing Standard* 13 (9): 45–7.

Mardell, A., and Rees, C. (1998). 'The theatre nurse: getting the image right.' *Nursing Standard* 13 (4): 46–7.

McColgan, K. (2006). 'Increasing surgical throughput in a busy day procedure unit.' *Journal of Perioperative Practice* 16 (2): 95–100.

McCulloch, J. (1998). 'Infection control: principles for practice.' *Nursing Standard.* 13 (1): 49–56.

Montgomery, J. (2003). *Health Care Law.* 2nd Edition. Oxford: Oxford University Press.

Moroney, N., and Knowles, C.H. (2006). 'Innovation and teamwork: introducing multidisciplinary team ward rounds.' *Nursing Management* **13** (1): 28–31.

NHS Estates (1998). *Health Technical Memorandum 2025: Ventilation in Healthcare Premises*. London: HMSO.

NHS Institute for Innovation and Improvement (2005). *Improvement Leaders Guide: Process Mapping, Analysis and Redesign*. London: DoH Publications.

NHS Litigation Authority (2008). *NHSLA Risk Management Standards for Acute Trusts*. London: NHSLA.

NICE (2004). *The Assessment and Prevention of Falls in Older People*. London: HMSO.

NICE (2006). *Patient safety and reduction of risk of transmission of Creutzfeldt-Jakob disease (CJD) via interventional procedures*. London: HMSO.

NICE (2008). *Ranibizumab and pegaptanib for the treatment of age-related macular degeneration*. London: HMSO.

Nursing and Midwifery Council (2008). The Code: Standards of Conduct, Performance and Ethics for Nurses and Midwives. London: NMC.

Pisani, S. (2004). 'Fibres found during cataract surgery.' *British Journal of Perioperative Nursing* **14** (11): 508–14.

Price, B. (2006). 'Exploring person-centred care.' *Nursing Standard* **20** (50): 49–56.

Rees, C. (1999). 'Brave new world.' *Nursing Standard* **14** (4): 43–4.

Reveley, S., Walsh, M., and Carlisle, A. (2002). 'Setting up a nurse practitioner service.' *Nursing Standard* **17** (10): 33–7.

Rogers, M., and Taylor, R. (2007). 'Counting the cost as Payment by Results changes healthcare funding in the NHS.' *Nursing Management* **14** (1): 8–11.

Royal College of Nursing (2005). *Maxi Nurses: Nurses Working in Advanced and Extended Roles Promoting and Developing Patient-centred Health Care*. London: RCN.

Royal College of Ophthalmologist (2008). *UK Vision Strategy launched to 'address inequalities' which lead to unnecessary blindness*. Online, available from: http://www.rcophth.ac.uk/docs/press/VISION2020FINAL.doc (accessed 30 April 2008).

Scott, E., and Summerball, L. (2004). 'Managing risk in the perioperative environment.' *Nursing Standard* **18** (30): 47–52.

Tingle, J. (2002). 'An introduction to clinical negligence: nurses and the law.' *British Journal of Nursing* **11** (15): 1033–5.

Wadsworth, L., Smith, A., and Waterman, H. (2002). 'The nurse practitioner's role in day case pre-operative assessment.' *Nursing Standard* **16** (47): 41–4.

Westwood, F. (2001). *Achieving Best Practice: Shaping Professionals for Success*. London: McGraw-Hill.

Wilson, J., and Bunnell, T. (2007). 'A review of the merits of the nurse practitioner role.' *Nursing Standard* **21** (18): 35–40.

WHO (1994). *A Declaration on the Promotion of the Patient's Rights in Europe*. Available on-line from: http://www.who.int/genomics/public/eu_declaration1994.pdf. Accessed June 2007.

WHO (2005). *State of the World's Sight. Vision 2020:the Right to Sight 1999–2005*. Executive Summary. Geneva: WHO.

Xavier, G. (1999). 'Asepsis.' *Nursing Standard* **13** (36): 49–53.

Chapter 7

Legal and ethical issues in ophthalmic nursing

Paul Buka

Ethics and the clinical relationship in ophthalmic nursing
  a) **Ethics and the four principles (Principlism)**
Sources of law
Duty of care applied to ophthalmic nursing
Organ donation and the law
  a) **The statutory provisions in ophthalmic, practice including: Corneal Tissue Act 1986, Human Tissue Act 1961, Human Organ Transplant Act 1989 (& regulations)**
Implications of employment law
  a) **Health and Safety Legislation & the Health and Safety at Work Act 1974, and the duties under sections 1 and 2.**
  b) **Vicarious liability**
  c) **Professional accountability**
  d) **Elements of informed consent**
Duty of confidentiality and record keeping
The patient's human rights and the law

Introduction

The preceding chapter considers an important level of clinical aspects of ophthalmic nursing in theatres. This is about clinical relationships which are important from the ethical and legal perspectives as the patient is more vulnerable in a theatre environment due to clinical needs. Nurses therefore need to be aware of this in light of not only their professional responsibilities but also the patient's corresponding rights. This chapter aims to give the reader an overview of current legal and ethical aspects of clinical practice in general and, in particular, ophthalmic nursing, as well as the opportunity to apply the relevant principles. There are always professional implications for clinical practice and for nurses. These are underpinned by the NMC Professional Code: Standards of conduct, performance and ethics for nurses and midwives (2008). Current inter-professional working provisions have seen nurse practitioners take on increasingly autonomous and extended roles, and also face not only new challenges but also new responsibilities. In ophthalmic nursing, as in any other specialist nursing discipline, it is now (more than ever) necessary for the practitioner to ensure their awareness not only of current research but also of any current ethical debate and law. In practice they may face what could be a potential minefield in disciplinary action, litigation and/or criminal prosecution. Currently, nurses can now assume an extended role as an autonomous practitioner in areas previously practised rather by the ophthalmologist, in areas such as Accidents and Emergency, involving procedures such as biometry, visual fields and pre- assessments for cataracts. Ongoing case law developments affecting the ophthalmic nurse include cases like the Alder Hey and Bristol. With all their advantages, professional advancement and personal development unfortunately come at a price – therefore it is important that the nurse is equipped for such new challenges. Current law as well as the professional code of conduct regulate the parameters within which a healthcare professional is expected to operate. It is therefore important that the nurse follows evidence-based practice, to support their conduct (Dale, 2006).

No citizen is above the law and this applies equally to practitioners as well as to hospital managers, when patient care is implemented. Sometimes when a conflict of interests arises, it may be necessary to seek a judicial review by the courts. A case of a professional who fails to comply with professional standards may result in professional disciplinary action and more. As an employee, a nurse's negligent act may also be a breach of the terms of a contract of employment that results in disciplinary action. This may also result in employment law, professional conduct disciplinary actions, as well as either prosecution or litigation by an injured patient or their representatives.

Ethics and the clinical relationship in ophthalmic nursing

Ethics and the clinical relationship

The customs and morality of a given society play a crucial role in shaping its ethical values, which may be imported into professional practice. No matter how morally reprehensible breach of an ethical principle may seem to most people, there is no automatic recognition by the law which would result in prosecution or litigation. Ethical or moral values must also inevitably underpin professional healthcare practice. Established ethical frameworks are respected by healthcare professionals and may influence management of ethical dilemmas arising in the delivery of care. Ethical principles however do not have the force of law. The study of morality, sometimes known as Moral Philosophy or Ethics, is concerned with right and wrong when it comes to human actions:

> Ethics is about moral choices. It is about the values that lie behind them, the reasons people give for them…it is about innocence and guilt, right and wrong and what it means to live a good or bad life…dilemmas of life, death…
>
> (Thompson, 2000, p. 1)

Ethics has also been described as, 'the rational discussion of that [decision making] process' (Thompson, 2003, p. 1). When faced with a dilemma, professionals should first look to their own code of conduct for guidance. Clinical judgements may also be influenced by the individual professional's ethical beliefs, based on their societal, cultural and/or religious background. These are core ethical principles, which though they do not have the force of law, have gained respect in most clinical situations, for example the universally accepted concept that it is wrong to unjustifiably kill another person.

> Whether a society has an ethical system can be recognised by its having a mental construct of values which are expressed as principles to be invoked and interpreted in guiding social behaviour (i.e. that which has meaning for

others) and in judging it in gradations of good or bad.

(Silberbauer, 2003, p. 17)

Moral dilemmas often arise when the patient lacks capacity for informed consent (which is discussed below), as addressed in the Mental Capacity Act 2005 (effective from October 2007). The relationship between a healthcare professional and their client is a therapeutic one, based on trust. The patient is therefore entitled to privacy, as enshrined in Article 8 of the Human Rights Act 1998.

When clinicians make clinical decisions, while advocating for their patient and acting in the patient's best interests, this should be based on their professional code of conduct, going beyond mere personal moral convictions.

Ethics and the four principles

Principlism is one healthcare ethical framework, commonly used across disciplines. Beauchamp and Childress (2004) added the first principle to the three-principle framework (below) which is said to have originated from Hippocrates. The four principles have now become an important part of medical/nursing ethics. These are common to all caring professions providing '...a common basic analytical framework and a common basic moral language' (Gillon, 1994, p. 1). Principlism consists of the following principles:

1. Autonomy

2. Beneficence

3. Non-maleficence

4. Fairness or justice

Respect for patient autonomy

This is the most important principle, being central to the delivery of care. A patient who is legally competent to make an informed choice can only be said to be in control of their present treatment and future welfare when they are given the opportunity to exercise this right. They have the right to accept or refuse treatment. The Patient's Charter (DoH, 1996, a policy statement) was seen as a catalyst for the debate on patient empowerment and patient rights. Patient autonomy is therefore:

The right of patients to make decisions about their medical care, without their health care provider trying to influence the decision. Patient autonomy does allow for health care providers to educate the patient but does not allow the health care provider to make the decision for the patient.

(Webster's New World Medical Dictionary, 2nd edition, 2003)

An example is that of parents of a child diagnosed with bilateral Retinoblastoma making an informed choice to have another baby. Another example involves a patient with acute chemical burns who, having been made aware of the risks involved, refuses to have eye irrigation.

At the other end of the spectrum, the paternalistic view held that the doctor and to some extent, other healthcare professionals, had the 'all-knowing' capacity to advocate for what they judged to be in their patient's best interests.

The post war National Health Service (NHS) Act 1946 may be seen as having raised the level of the general public's expectations, of 'a seamless service', which would care for people from 'cradle to grave'. In light of limited resources, this may now be unrealistic and have to be modified. The caring process may at times be dogged with controversy and difficulties when conflicts of interests arise. The interests of healthcare service providers may be pitched against those of patients as service users and their representatives. Expectations do not always match (Thompson, 2003). Others take a dim view of the nature of caring relationships and have no doubt as to whose interests are paramount; 'there can be little doubt that health care professionals are imposing "treatment" on patients which cannot be shown to be exclusively in the patient's interest' (Brazier, 2003, p. 109). Patient autonomy may not be achievable when dealing with a patient who lacks the capacity to consent, for example, where children or vulnerable adults are concerned. Section 1 of the Mental Capacity Act 2005 requires an assessment of a patient's capacity based on five principles:

1. A person must be assumed to have capacity unless it is established that he lacks capacity.

2. A person is not to be treated as unable to make a decision unless all practicable steps to help him to do so have been taken without success.

3. A person is not to be treated as unable to make a decision merely because he makes an unwise decision.

4. An act done, or decision made, under this Act for or on behalf

of a person who lacks capacity must be done, or made, in his best interests.

5. Before the act is done, or the decision is made, regard must be had to whether the purpose for which it is needed can be as effectively achieved in a way that is less restrictive of the person's rights and freedom of action.

Beneficence

All the actions of the healthcare professional must promote good or enhance some benefits for the patient under their care. The professional is expected to intervene through decisions which are in the patient's best interests and promote their welfare. This also relates to the duty of care (the law of tort), not to harm patients through actions or omissions. This will be explored further below.

Non-maleficence

This principle requires avoidance of bad or negative conduct that may cause harm to the patient and to others. Section 7 of the Health and Safety at Work Act, 1974, covers this area. This is also about avoiding any negative actions or omissions that may cause harm to the patient. The principle is related to the common law concept of avoiding omissions (under both English and Scots Law) and the duty of care to a patient, e.g. patients' needs should be addressed adequately, by avoiding unnecessary and risky delays in an inefficient triage system in Accident and Emergency (A&E).

Justice or fairness

Justice considers the ability to consider options, based on fairness, aiming to achieve a balanced outcome in the face of competing interests. The clinician should treat all their patients with the respect and fairness they deserve. Their decisions should be influenced by clinical need but they must balance their clinical decisions against the practicality of available resources. This may be difficult to achieve when limited resources for care are considered. For example, patients who lack the knowledge or ability to access information on their care should be treated fairly.

It is fair to say that some legal obligations may be informed by morality. Ethics on the other hand, does not necessarily have to be justified by or be based on legal principles. More importantly, there are professional ethical standards governing the conduct of healthcare professionals. The law may be called upon to intervene, as and when necessary, in clinical decisions (Mason *et al.*, 2002).

Sources of law

Sources
of law

The United Kingdom (UK) law (unlike countries like France where the law is codified) derives from a variety of sources, which include the following:

- *International Treaties.* These are agreed mostly through world organisations and states, such as the United Nations, and are adopted by signatory countries across the world. An example is the United Nations Conventions on Refugees 1951.

- *The European Union* (EU) law has introduced new elements into UK law. Since accession to the Treaty of Rome 1957, most aspects of the above law bind all United Kingdom subjects (unless they are part of opted out aspects). Otherwise EU legislation now takes precedence over the national parliament and all of the parliaments of the four UK countries, subject to s2 (1) European Community Act 1972: any '...rights created by or arising out of the community treaties shall have effect on UK Law' (McHale *et al.*, 1998, p. 8). The provisions of the treaty are amended as time progresses; one example is the new Lisbon Treaty signed in 2007. There are two main types of EU legislation:

  a) Directives – these are laws passed from the European Parliament and, subject to member states implementing them through their own national legislation by an agreed time table.

  b) Regulations – these are EU laws which must be applied by member states in their entirety.

- *The UK Parliament:* There are also aspects of European law, which do not apply, subject to the United Kingdom (UK) government exercising its rights to opt out, which means that its citizens would not be bound by such provisions.

- *Common/Judge-made law.* Sometimes called case law, this is the most common type of law, which is found in judgements in cases, which have come before the courts as judges interpret the intention of the legislators and apply the law at different levels. A decision in a higher Court of Law, which sets a 'precedent' has more authority than a lower one and must be followed by the latter. (A precedent is an established legal principle or decision, which in turn binds lower courts, which are obliged to follow it.) An English court is however not bound by a decision from a Scottish or other court following the Common Law. It may find such decisions 'persuasive' in reaching its own conclusion if no English court decision exists. A decision by the House of Lords binds any lower courts within the United Kingdom.

● *Byelaws and Delegated legislation.* These are derived from Enabling or Parent acts and are created through government ministers and devolved authority assigned to bodies like local authorities and quasi-autonomous non-governmental organisations (QUANGOs). The problem with this group of legislation is that it is more open to abuse, for example by local authorities acting 'ultra vires' or beyond the scope of their powers. This can however be challenged for clarification of the intention of parliament, in a court of law.

Laws are usually recognisable because they are universal to all citizens to whom they are addressed, though they may apply to a specific group or class of people. They should also be promulgated or published in order to be applicable to citizens. Laws usually define rights as well as create obligations with commensurate sanctions. They are necessary in order to create harmony and to ensure justice and fairness to all. As a basic tenet, it is been argued in the courts that it is a key principle that no citizen should be above the law.

Duty of care applied to ophthalmic nursing

Duty of care

Duty of care is a term, which has a moral basis. It is the source of our obligations towards others with whom we may have a relationship. This reinforces the need to check medication before application to patient, such as being aware of and acting on relevant factors like contraindications and expiry date, for example, avoiding instillation of eye drops contraindicated for a patient who also suffers from asthma. The following definition is generally accepted as a foundation in Tort Law:

> '...you must take reasonable care to avoid acts or omissions which you can reasonably foresee would be likely to injure your neighbour.' Ld Atkins, at p. 580, *Donaghue v Stevenson* HL 1932, All ER Rep1.

> The claimant had visited a café with a friend, who had bought her some ice cream and a drink of ginger beer, the café owner poured some of the drink over her ice cream, and she consumed it. When she poured the rest of the contents of the bottle, she found the decomposing remains of a dead snail. The claimant became unwell as a result, she could however not claim against the seller, as she had no contract with him. Instead, she successfully brought a claim for negligence (in Tort) against the manufacturer. The courts recognised the manufacturer's duty of care to the consumer.

The court took the view that a manufacturer who allows a defective product to leave their possession for distribution for sale owes a duty of care to its ultimate consumer. In response to the question 'who is my neighbour', the House of Lords established the so-called 'neighbour principle' in the above case:

> ...Persons who are so closely affected by my act that I ought reasonably to have them in my contemplation as being affected when I am directing my mind to the acts or omissions which are called in question
> Ld Atkins, at p. 580, *Donaghue v Stevenson* 1932, HL All ER Rep1

The question of duty of care may arise when there is an allegation of negligence, and where care is said to have fallen below certain specific standards. Due to their special relationship, there is usually little difficulty in establishing that a healthcare professional who is responsible for treating a patient owes them a duty of care not to harm them as well as to avoid omissions, which may cause them (patients) any harm. An example of breach of duty of care is if a nurse administers eye drops to a patient knowing them to have a known allergy to them. This is the applied principle of the 'Donaghue' case, above.

The Law of Tort, which deals with claims in damages for personal injury, has certain pre-requisites before an injured party can raise an action for damages for personal injuries in Tort Law.

They are called 'hurdles' which need to be overcome before a claim is successful. These usually require the following order:

1. That the claimant is owed *a duty of care* by the particular respondent. This is to prevent unwarranted and frivolous claims which may be unrelated to the alleged injury before the court.

2. A *breach of that duty by the respondent* must be established by the victim. There must be a sufficient degree of proximity in their relationship.

3. The claimant suffered *harm as a result of the alleged breach.*

4. Did the alleged breach cause the harm in question? – Was it a *causal nexus* in the chain of causation?

5. There is reasonable foreseeability (on the part of the defendant/respondent) pertaining to *limitation of damages.* This means that the defendant has limited liability.

The law is subsequently developed in the more recent case of *Caparo Industries v. Dickman [1990] 2 AC 605* which is currently the leading case on negligence and duty of care. The principles which are often applied to healthcare cases require that the following 'three-fold test' be applied before a victim's claim can succeed:

● harm must be a 'reasonably foreseeable' result of the defendant's conduct

● a relationship of 'proximity' between the defendant and the claimant

● it must be 'fair, just and reasonable' to impose liability.
   (Caparo Industries v. Dickman [1990] 2 AC 605)

The most common claim in a personal injury case is for 'negligence' and the time limit for this is normally three years under the Limitations Act 1980 or the Prescription and Limitation (Scotland) Act 1973. The effect is that court proceedings must be issued within three years of the victim first being aware of having suffered an injury. A victim claiming damages must also establish (on a balance of probabilities) the above hurdles before the courts can award damages for personal injury in Tort (McHale *et al.*, 1998). Some claims fall short of the requirements at the initial hurdles as it can be difficult to prove clinical negligence at times, especially where there are latent complications of a clinical event, which may surface a long time after this happens.

There are different time limits within which a victim must

begin legal action in a personal injury claim. For deliberately caused personal injury, however, the limitation period is 6 years from the date of injury. Latent claims may be allowed at the discretion of the court. Litigation is usually an uphill struggle and most victims cannot afford the hassle, the time, and money to fight a case. In order to recover damages, a Claimant must establish on a balance of probabilities that the Defendant's negligence had a material affect on the outcome of the disease. For healthcare professionals who hold themselves out as having a specialist skill, they will be judged by the standards of a reasonably competent healthcare professional, which are higher standards than the most basic. The standard of care expected by the courts is that of the 'reasonable' clinician, which is the higher rather than the lower one, what is called the 'Bolam Standards', this is based on the Bolam v Friern Hospital Management Committee [1957] 1 WLR 583 (discussed below) The following case developed these standards further:

> *Wilsher v Essex Area Health Authority (1987)* QB 730.CA, 1988 AC 1074 HL 1988 1 All ER 87

> The Claimant was born prematurely. Subsequently the Defendant negligently gave the Claimant excess oxygen. A catheter was wrongly inserted into his vein on two occasions instead of his artery and as a result, he developed an incurable eye condition. The court accepted that although his blindness could have been caused by one of any other conditions found in premature babies. The hospital admitted only negligence in general on that basis but the court upheld the objective standard in respect of a junior doctor who could not argue his inexperience as a reason to avoid liability. The Hospital was found to be negligent and damages were awarded.

Davies (2001) acknowledges that there may be difficulties in accessing evidence which is mainly in medical records. The reality of the matter is that over many years, witnesses may move, forget what happened, or may die before the case comes to court. Delays may also disadvantage a patient. The Data Protection Act 1998 gives a patient or their representative a right to access clinical records. It is therefore important to maintain accurate record keeping. There may be difficulties in a case where say, a nurse administered first aid without making a record of this and subsequently, the patient's condition deteriorated.

Organ donation and the law

Organ donation and the law

The Human Tissue Act 1961 and the Human Organ Transplant Act 1989 have been the mainstay legislation (in all the four countries of the United Kingdom) for this area for some time until the recent introduction of the Human Tissue Act 2004. This statute has repealed the above legislation in England and Wales and Northern Ireland and repealed it in part in Scotland. Current provisions require that:

> The person lawfully in possession of the body of a deceased person [for our purposes the doctor or other person designated on behalf of the hospital] may authorise the removal of any part from the body for the use for therapeutic purposes or for purposes of medical education or research if [indicating a condition or that what follows must be satisfied] having made such reasonable enquiry as may be practicable…he has no reason to believe that …any surviving relative of the deceased objects to the body being so dealt with.
>
> (Section 1(3) of the Human Tissue Act 1961)

There are however some difficulties, e.g. where a corneal transplant is used, there may be issues of some risk of conditions such as Creutzfeldt-Jakob disease (CJD). There has been some Department of Health (DoH) clarification on the need for the person in possession of the body to ensure the relatives do not object to removal of tissue (HSC (IS) 156 Guidance circular to NHS Authorities, 1975).

Implications of employment law

Employment law

Employment law regulates the conditions and relationship and the behaviour between the employer and an employee in the workplace (Sargeant, 2001). The employer is also required by section 2 of the Health and Safety at Work Act 1974 (HSWA 1974), not only to carry out risk assessments, but also has a duty of care (section 1 of the above statute) to ensure that people who come into their premises are safe. The employee likewise, is bound by section 7 of the same statute to ensure their own reasonable safety and that of others. Since this statute, both these parties are now required to avoid harmful actions or omissions, by removing hazards and minimising risk in the workplace depending on the likelihood and magnitude of the risk. One example is where a partially sighted patient is allowed to use a hot water tap where they may be scalded.

As professionals, nurses are reminded that they are personally accountable for actions and omissions in their practice (NMC, 2008). This includes nurses on specialist ophthalmic wards as well as other healthcare professionals providing acute and primary care.

Vicarious liability in employment

An employer is expected to profit or benefit from the input and positive outcomes of their employees. The employer has a legal responsibility to issue terms and conditions of service within two months of employment (Du Feu and Warnock, 1995). Accordingly, the employer should bear the liability or loss resulting from any negligent actions of their employees, for example, a nurse applying an eye patch too firmly with resulting loss of vision. The usual presumption in employment law is that the employer has overall or ultimate responsibility for the actions which are carried out by the employee 'in the course of their employment'. The nature of this relationship raises questions as to who should take responsibility for the wrongful actions of employees. Given that as the employer is responsible for the actions of their employees (carried out in the course of their employment) they are therefore the ultimate beneficiary of the positive actions of their employees, correspondingly the employer is taken to be responsible for the negative actions of their employees. The general rule therefore is that whoever has control of hiring and firing, setting out the terms and conditions of service or ground rules and paying the wages has liability for any negligent actions of employees. There have however been conflicting employment law decisions on this issue in the courts.

There are two of types of employment contracts, namely:

(a) *a contract of services*, which is the normal agreement to work under agreed terms for a specific wage or salary – most employees work under such a contract and this should be a written contract, though in dispute, verbal contracts can be proved through the conduct of the two parties.

(b) *a contract for services* – this applies to agency or hired workers who are either self-employed through an agency or working for themselves.

Vicarious liability is usually presumed in the first instance, provided the act was arrived out 'in the course of their employment'. The position is not quite as clear cut in the 'contract for services', though some cases have gone against the employer based on the 'agency principle' in Contract Law. If however, an employee acts illegally or outside the scope of their work, the question arises whether the employer would still be vicariously liable. The point in issue is illustrated by the case of *Lister and Others v Hall (2001) UK, HL, 22*. A warden who was an employee at a boarding school to look after young boys, instead abused them. The court held that although the defendant carried out criminal acts, which were not authorised by his employer, this was nevertheless, 'in the course of his employment' and therefore the employer was liable under vicarious liability.

One argument in favour of suing the employer is that there is an assumption that the employer is a better financial position to bear the cost of litigation. The employer nevertheless has a right to recompense any losses from a negligent healthcare employee. In practice most healthcare professionals are indemnified by insurance for any mishaps.

Professional accountability

Professional accountability relates to answerability or the readiness to give an explanation or justification for one's actions or omissions to interested parties. This includes the patient, the regulatory body, the NMC, professional colleagues, as well as the law. Clearly due to the principle of accountability, a healthcare professional may not hide behind an employer's vicarious liability because they '...are accountable for the actions they take as well as their omissions' (Fletcher and Buka, 1999, p. 54). An example is in a case of day surgery for a cataract operation, a nurse must ensure good practice and that hospital procedure and policy is followed at all times. Unqualified staff on the other hand, are usually said to be responsible for their actions as they are not answerable to a professional body. When judging whether a nurse acted below the expected standard a court of law will need to ask whether, in acting in the way they did, they were acting in accordance with a practice of competent respected professional opinion (Bolam Standard). The Bolam standard is applied thus, '...the test is the standard of the ordinary competent man [or woman] exercising and professing to have that special skill...' (from Mc Nair, J.'s judgement (1957) in the following case:

> a patient suffering from endogenous depression was undergoing electric convulsive therapy. He sustained injury and multiple fractures during shock treatment, having not had a muscle relaxant administered. He sued for personal injury. It was held that the action was entitled to fail if the professionals could show that in exercising reasonable care in carrying out the treatment they had followed a set of procedures (policies), backed by a professional body even if there was another body of opinion with a contrary view.
>
> Bolam v Frien Hospital Management Committee [1957] 1 WLR 582

The problem with the above approach however is that there can be difficulties when dealing with self-regulating professionals like doctors. They set their own standards with possible accusations of 'covering each other's backs' while purportedly protecting the patient. The following case clarified Bolam:

> A case of a child where a doctor failed to put a tube down the throat of a child to assist his breathing. Five experts said that the doctor had been negligent and three said she had not. Lord Browne-Wilkinson ruled that only in very rare cases should a judge reject the evidence of a professional expert as being 'unreasonable', but he was entitled to do so.
>
> Bolitho v City and Hackney Health Authority [1997] 3 WLR 582

In the above case, majority expert evidence was admitted and influenced the decision of the court, thus establishing the principle that it was at times necessary for the court to go beyond the expertise of the alternative practitioner. The courts also must have regard to the fact that a practitioner was practicing their skills based on what is generally accepted as standard practice.

Levels of accountability therefore, are to the patient, professional colleagues through the professional body, the employer and to the law of the land.

Elements of informed consent

The basic principle of consent is that every person has a right to choose what should be done with his or her body. The elements of consent are that it:

- must be given voluntarily
- must be given by a competent person
- is informed to a sufficient degree of information(UKCC (2002), paragraphs 3.3 and 3.4).

Other essential elements which should be considered include a patient's ability to understand and retain information relating to their ophthalmic treatment as well as their ability to make an informed choice on treatment. One example in ophthalmic practice is the pre-assessment area of practice. On admission for a cataract operation, a patient may consent to a procedure without understanding whether this would be under a general or local anaesthetic. All patients have a common law right to give or withhold consent on treatment, which the Department of Health (DoH) (2001b) recognises. Overriding consent may be tantamount to client abuse, and in breach of Article 3 of the Human Rights Act 1998. This may also amount to the criminal act of assault. There are however exceptions to the rule when a patient lacks the capacity to consent.

Consent to treatment may be explicit, implicit (implied), verbal or written. Further exceptions to the rule are: emergencies – when the clinicians are expected always to act in the patient's best interests. Such is the case for incapacitated patients, e.g. consent for emergency surgery when two consultants may consent to an operation on behalf of such a patient. In the case of children however, the minimum age for consent is 16, under the so-called Gillick or 'Fraser' Competence, in Gillick v West Norfolk and Wisbech Area Health Authority and another HL, [1986] 1 AC 112. The implications of this case were to allow children younger than 16 who are deemed to have a sufficient degree of understanding, to make a decision to accept treatment.

Subject to the Mental Capacity Act 2005, and the Adults with

Incapacity (Scotland Act (2004), healthcare advocates may be appointed to act as proxy and make decisions on behalf of the incapacitated patient. The significance of a donor card is that it is recognised as evidence of a patient's presumed consent for use of body tissue including corneal tissue. It is also helpful if a potential donor has communicated their wishes to family members. Any person can sign up to the NHS Donor UK Transplant. A patient who is under the age of 16 would be free under the law governing informed consent to express their wishes to donate corneal tissue if they have a sufficient degree of understanding to be considered competent to make such a decision and guardians agree.

Since the case of *Airedale N.H.S. Trust-v-Bland* (1993) 2 WLR 316, (the Tony Bland case) English Common Law now provides that, 'Advance Directives' may be drawn up (under the ordinary rules of drawing up a will) in the form of a Living Will. This may be taken into consideration in establishing the wishes of the patient. Power of attorney and court of protection advocacy does not involve treatment decisions as these involve representation of the patient's property rights interests.

THINKING POINT

Ms A, aged 60, lives alone in a terraced house, with a past ophthalmic history of retinal detachment in one eye and bilateral Primary Open Angle Glaucoma (POAG). She has had to undergo surgery for detachment.

On this admission, she was due to have a vitrectomy. She underwent surgery the next day and was discharged home the following day. On discharge, the consultant advised the patient to remain in bed in the same position for at least a week and probably up to 6–8 weeks (and return for a check up within a week).

The clinicians were aware that on discharge, the patient would have a 70-mile journey by car. The verbal advice was for her to keep her head in the same position – tipped downwards while sitting upright. She was also told that she would need another person to stay with her for a week. *continued overleaf*

There were no arrangements made for any district nurse follow up or other care and no documented evidence of a discharge plan. The patient did however make her own arrangements for private domestic help. On the basis of the information she was given it meant that she would have to spend time in the indicated upright position for approximately 70–80% of her time. She found it extremely difficult to comply with these instructions during the post recovery period.

One of several things could have gone wrong.

1. What are the ethical, legal and professional issues in this case?

2. What legal rights would the patient have should things go wrong?

Duty of confidentiality and record keeping

Duty of confidentiality

The Caldicott Report 1997, on personally-identifiable information, recommended that 'Guardians' of personal information be appointed, whose main function would be to safeguard, monitor the use and quality of confidential information within NHS organisation (DoH, 2001b). Caldicott principles and processes provide a framework of quality standards for the management of confidentiality and access to personal information under the leadership of a Caldicott guardian (DoH, 2001b, p. 2):

Principle 1 – Justify the purpose.

Principle 2 – Don't use patient-identifiable information unless it is absolutely necessary

Principle 3 – Use the minimum necessary patient-identifiable information.

Principle 4 – Access to patient-identifiable information should be on a strict need-to-know basis.

Principle 5 – Everyone with access to patient-identifiable information should be aware of their responsibilities.

Principle 6 – Understand and comply with the law.

The Data Protection Act 1998 regulates access to information that is held electronically, including the obtaining and storage of data. It is important that national standards have been set for record keeping and all NHS records are public records under the terms of the Public Records Act 1958 S.3 (1)-(2). Some of the reasons why healthcare practitioners need accurate patient records include:

● to support patient care and continuity of care

● to support evidence-based clinical practice

● to support sound administrative and managerial decision making, as part of the knowledge base for NHS services

● to meet legal requirements, including requests from patients under access to health records legislation

● to assist medical and other audits

● to support improvements in clinical effectiveness through research (DoH, 1999, p. 4).

The basis of the clinical relationship is said to be a privileged one for the clinician, who has access to confidential information relating to a patient. The patient on the other hand is generally in a vulnerable position. The duty of confidentiality is one of the important implied terms in Employment Law. Due to the way confidential information is acquired by the nurse, it is unethical for the nurse to unlawfully disclose confidential information. An example is where a patient, who is seen with a red painful eye diagnosed as uveitis, turns out to be HIV positive and informs the nurse that they do not want other patients to be informed of this fact. This is a reasonable request and the nurse is required to ensure that this is the case.

There are however some exceptions when the law allows confidentiality to be breached if necessary in order to protect the general public, e.g. Public Health Act 1984. The circumstances in which a nurse may be required to breach that confidence are defined by law (Mason *et al.*, 2002; NMC, 2008). There are always dangers where information may be shared with other healthcare teams (Venereal Disease Act 1974 and National Health Service (VD) Regulations of 1974). In normal circumstances, genito-urinary clinics (like all other nursing areas) are bound by the Data Protection Act 1998, for confidentiality of clinical records. In both English and Scottish law, the patient's right to privacy is safeguarded by human rights law and the confidentiality requirement, except in certain circumstances, as defined by the law (Mason *et al.*, 2002). It is nevertheless a mandatory requirement for healthcare professionals to report specific infectious diseases under the Public Health (Control of Disease) Act 1984 and the Public Health (Infectious Diseases) Regulations 1988.

The aim of a regulated breach is the protection of the general public.

The patient's human rights and the law

Human rights and the law

The Human Rights Act 1998 received Royal Assent on 9 November 1998 (Leckie and Pickergill, 2000, p. 1). Since 2 October 2001, public authorities have a duty to safeguard individual rights and these can be enforced in UK courts. Judges have the power to refer to parliament for clarification of the intention of legislature, if the law is uncertain. Some of the important aspects of human rights which may affect practice are as follows:

Article 2

Everyone's right to life shall be protected by law. No one shall be deprived of his life intentionally save in the execution of a sentence of a court following his conviction of a crime for which this penalty is provided by law.

Article 3 – prohibition of torture

No one shall be subjected to torture or inhuman or degrading treatment or punishment.

An example of an alleged breach of this article was the following case:

> *NHS Trust A v M and NHS Trust B v H* [2001] Fam 348 where a hospital sought permission to discontinue artificial hydration and nutrition to a person, who had been diagnosed as being in a 'permanent vegetative state'. The Court noted that Article 2 imposed a positive obligation to give treatment where that is in the best interests of the patient – but not where it would be futile. Discontinuing treatment would not be an intentional deprivation of life under Article 2; and provided that withdrawing treatment was in line with a respected body of medical opinion and that the patient would be unaware of the treatment and not suffering, there would be no breach of his right to be free of

inhuman or degrading treatment under Article 3.

http://www.dh.gov.uk/en/Managingyourorganisation/Equalityandhumanrights/Humanrights/DH_4136019

Article 8 – right to respect for private and family life

1. Everyone has the right to his private and family life, his home and his correspondence.

2. There shall be no interference by a public authority with the exercise of this right except such as is in accordance with the law.

This is consistent with the patient's right of autonomy, consent to treatment and informed choice.

Article 17 – prohibition of abuse of rights

Nothing in this Convention may be interpreted as implying for any State, group or person any right to engage in any activity or perform any act aimed at the destruction of any of the rights and freedoms set forth herein or at their limitation to a greater extent than is provided for in the Convention.

Current legislation is underpinned by the Human Tissue Act 2004. Its main aim was:

> …to provide a consistent legislative framework for issues relating to whole body donation and the taking, storage and use of human organs and tissue. It will make consent the fundamental principle underpinning the lawful storage and use of human bodies, body parts, organs and tissue and the removal of material from the bodies of deceased persons. It will set up an over-arching authority which is intended to rationalize existing regulation of activities like transplantation and anatomical examination,… It is intended to achieve a balance between the rights and expectations of individuals and families, and broader considerations…

> (Human Tissue Act 2004, Explanatory Notes (4))

The relevant legislation that is repealed by this statute is as follows:

- The Corneal Tissue Act 1986 (c. 18), which deals with the removal of eyes
- The Human Tissue Act 1961 (c. 54)
- The Anatomy Act 1984 (c. 14).

In principle, doctors could overrule any relatives' objection, (HSC (IS) 156 Guidance Circular to NHS Authorities; Human Tissue Act,

1961). The Human Organ Transplant Act 1989 (c. 31) outlawed commercial dealing of organs (from outside the United Kingdom) for transplant.

Conclusion

When the Human Tissue Act of 1961 was passed one of its aims included the provision for acquiring consent from relatives (where they were available) before the removal of eyes for corneal grafts. The lessons learnt from the cases of unauthorised removal of human organs such as eyes, without consent mean that such instances of abuse should not be repeated. There has been debate on calls for new legislation to allow 'presumed consent', which gives healthcare professionals the right to remove any body organs or tissue as they see fit unless there are objections.

The Human Tissue Act 2004 came into effect following the Alder Hey scandal and the public outcry, with '...An Act to make provision with respect to activities involving human tissue; to make provision about the transfer of human remains from certain museum collections; and for connected purposes.' The Human Tissue Act (2004) now has as its main aim to safeguard the consent of patients' next of kin, including partners of the deceased, with a wider definition and to '...enshrine consent as the clear basis for the keeping of tissue and organ' – (John Reid, 2003). It also gives the Secretary of State powers of entry and seizure of records of hospitals. The enhanced provisions for protection of 'appropriate' consent are contained in section 1 of the same act. Consent must be signed and attested by at least one witness. The statute also creates an offence punishable by a fine if no proper records are maintained. The legal position may yet be tested in a court of law as to what the likely outcome would be in the case where a relative raised an objection to a corneal donation in cases where the patient has a donor card.

The development of nursing and ophthalmic nursing as an important branch of the profession has meant that there are implications for practice involving the enhancement of the scope of professional practice with the relevant knowledge and skills informed by current law and ethical values. There is now a diversity of specialties all with an extended role and ophthalmic nursing is one such area. The consequence is better quality of care delivered within nursing in general and the specialist nurse roles in particular. There is now less dependence on the medical professionals within the nursing discipline as a whole. As practitioners, ophthalmic nurses are accountable for their own actions and omissions, and their knowledge of law and ethics will serve them well. One of the main issues facing nurses is how they respond to current and future challenges by equipping themselves with such knowledge on how to deal with nursing issues which affect them in their daily practice. The fact that values change within the law and ethics does impact ophthalmic practice as real and inevitable. The law especially evolves in response to the needs of society. The nurse has therefore responsibilities to ensure that they are up-to-date with current law and current professional ethical values.

This chapter considered the general principles in respect of the law and ethical values underpinning healthcare in ophthalmic nursing. Important issues are even more likely to surface when a vulnerable group of people such as children are subject to healthcare. The next chapter takes on board and analyses legal and ethical issues from the perspective of children in ophthalmic care. Due to their healthcare needs, any vulnerable persons, and more so children, should be offered a much higher level of protection. This is demonstrated by the development of specialised branches of law such as Child Law, which is applicable to this group of young persons; the general principles of law however remain the same. Ethical principles likewise often find common ground for all individuals receiving care, regardless of age or gender.

References

Beauchamp, T.L., and Childress, J. (2004). *Principles of Bioethics*. 5th edition. Oxford: Oxford University Press.

Brazier, M. (2003). *Medicine, Patients and the Law*. London: Penguin.

Dale, A.E. (2006). 'Determining guiding principles for evidence-based practice.' *Nursing Standard* 20 (25): 41–6.

Davies, M. (2001) *Textbook on Medical Law*. Blackstone Press.

Department of Health (1996). *The Patient's Charter and You*. London: Department of Health.

Department of Health (1999). Health Service Circular, HSC 1999/053.

Department of Health (2001a). *Implementing the Caldicott Standards into Social Care:* Consultation Paper on Caldicott Guardians. London: Department of Health. Available at www.dh.gov.uk (accessed 24 August 2008).

Department of Health (2001b).Caldicott Report (1997). The Department of Health Report on the review of patient-identifiable information © Crown Copyright 2001. Available at www.dh.gov.uk (accessed 24 August 2008).

Du Feu, V., and Warnock, O. (1995). *Employment Law in the NHS.* London: Cavendish Publishing Limited.

Fletcher, L., and Buka, P. (1999). *A Legal Framework for Caring.* Basingstoke: Palgrave Macmillan.

Gillon, R. (1994). 'Medical ethics: four principles plus attention to scope.' *British Medical Journal* 309: 184–8.

HSC (IS) 156 Guidance circular to NHS Authorities, (1975): Human Tissue Act, 1961. Available at www.dh.gov.uk/en/Publicationsandstatistics/Publications/PublicationsPolicyAndGuidance/Browsable/DH_4882861
(accessed 22 August 2008).

Leckie, D., and Pickersgill, D. (2000). *Human Rights Act Explained.* Norwich: The Stationery Office.

Mason, J., McCall, S., and Laurie, G. (2002). *Law and Medical Ethics.* London: Butterworths.

McHale, J., Tingle, J., and Peysner, J. (1998). *Law and Nursing.* Oxford: Butterworth Heinemann.

NMC (2008). Professional Code; *Standards of conduct, performance and ethics for nurses and midwives.* London: NMC.

Reid, J. (2003). 'Tissue "Theft" law unveiled.' Available at: http://news.bbc.co.uk/1/hi/health/3288955.stm, accessed 12 February 2008.

Sargeant, M. (2001). Employment Law. Harlow: Longman.

Silberbauer, G. (2003). *A Companion to Ethics.* Oxford: Blackwell Publishing.

Thompson, M. (2000). *Ethics.* London: Hodder and Stoughton.

UKCC (2002). *Guidelines for Records and Record Keeping.* London: NMC.

Webster's New World Medical Dictionary (2003). 2nd edition. Somerset: Wiley Publishing.
www.dh.gov.uk/en/Managingyourorganisation/Equalityandhumanrights/Humanrights/DH_4136019 (accessed 24 June 2006).

Statutes

Anatomy Act 1984

Corneal Tissue Act 1986

Data Protection Act 1998

European Community Act 1972

Health and Safety at Work Act 1974 (includes section7)

Healthcare Adults with Incapacity (Scotland) Act (2004)

Human Organ Transplant Act 1989

Human Rights Act 1998

Human Tissue Act 1961

Human Tissue Act 2004 © Crown copyright 2004

Limitations Act 1980

Lisbon Treaty 2007

Mental Capacity Act 2005

National Health Service Act 1946

National Health Service (VD) Regulations of 1974

Prescriptions and Limitations Act 1973

Public Health Act 1984

Public Health (Control of Disease) Act 1984

Public Health (Infectious Diseases) Regulations 1988

Public Records Act 1958

Treaty of Rome 1957

United Nations Conventions on Refugees 1951

Venereal Disease Act 1974

Cases

Airedale N.H.S. Trust v Bland (1993) 2 WLR 316

Bolam v Frien Hospital Management Committee (1957) 1 WLR 582

Bolitho v City and Hackney Health Authority (1997) 3 WLR 582

Caparo Industries v. Dickman (1990) 2 AC 605

Donaghue (or McAlister) v Stevenson (1932) All ER Rep 1; (1932)

Gillick v West Norfolk and Wisbech Area Health Authority and another HL (1986) 1 AC 112

Lister and Others v Hall (2001) UK, HL, 22

NHS Trust A v M and NHS Trust B v H (2001) Fam 348

Wilsher v Essex Area Health Authrity (1987) QB 730. A, 1988 AC 1074, HL 1988 1 All ER 87.

Chapter 8
Issues in paediatric ophthalmic nursing
Kathleen Chambers

Legal and ethical issues
Retinopathy of prematurity
National Service Framework for Children 2004
Protecting the vulnerable child
Handling disclosure information about child abuse

Introduction

As stated in Chapter 7 there are always legal and ethical implications for practitioners in clinical practice, but where children are concerned it has progressively become a potential minefield. Advanced technology in the areas of diagnosis, treatment and delivery of care afforded to children has a high impact on the role of the practitioner, especially the ophthalmic practitioner. There is therefore a need to understand the ethical and legal issues that surround children and be prepared to act on these issues when they arise, keeping in mind that the welfare of the child is paramount, as stated in the Children Act 1989. This chapter aims to give the reader insight into the current issues and future challenges of both ethical and legal decision making that face the practitioner within the fields of ophthalmic, general paediatrics, neonatal and midwifery practice, when providing care for children of all ages who have ocular conditions. This requires a sound professional knowledge and understanding of not only ophthalmic care but child care development and the law surrounding children.

Caring for children with ocular conditions is a growing area and it is not without its challenges and dilemmas for any practitioners providing health care. With the expansion of the National Health Service and private provision there are now children being treated in ophthalmic clinics by nurses who do not have training in paediatric specialities and children with eye injuries seen in paediatric clinics without the expertise of ophthalmic practitioners.

Legal and ethical issues

Legal and ethical issues

When the Children Act was enacted in 1989 it was seen as a major breakthrough in legislation regarding the care of children. The main focus was and still is that the 'best interest of the child is paramount'. However, since the introduction of the Human Rights Act 1998 this concept has been widely debated as giving children too many 'rights' to the detriment of their parents. In order to redress this there is now the Children Act 2004 and the appointment of a Children's Commissioner to oversee all aspects of child care in England. The Children Act 2004 has its focus on changes to the adoption law and looked after children; this may be why it has not had the impact that the Children Act 1989 had on practice. Under the UK Children Act (1989) a child is defined as any person under the age of 18 years. The 2004 Act has increased this age to 19 years and to 25 years if the child has a learning disability. This has had an impact on the future planning for the National Health Services and Social Care as now children will need to be seen under the requirements for paediatric services for longer. There is also an impact on where these children are admitted to, should they require inpatient treatment. Practitioners need also to be aware that these children are unique in the face of the law when suing for damages; unlike adults who have a maximum of three years, children have the right to sue for damages for any injury caused during their childhood until they reach their 19th birthday. This requires practitioners to think about what reports they need to write, how to write them and what information will be shared when they are working with other agencies. The two Acts now work in conjunction with each other and where changes have been made the 2004 Act now takes precedence. Many children are vulnerable to episodes of abuse from their so-called carers and this brings them into contact with the health service providers and admission into acute care at some time during their childhood. Practitioners now need to have a sound professional knowledge of both Acts in order to assess which is the appropriate one, the areas and classifications of abuse in order to distinguish between non-accidental injuries especially to the eyes and to be able to implement the correct procedures in order to safeguard the child from further injury.

The General Assembly of the United Nations (UN) adopted the Convention on the Rights of the Child in November 1989 and this was implemented into English law in January 1992. Linked to this is the Human Rights Act 1998 which came into effect in October 2000. These two Acts further highlight the potential of certain areas of health and social care practice which could affect the rights and freedoms which were promised under the Act. Article 3 of the Act refers to torture and degrading treatment or punishment; this has had an impact on child health practitioners especially when restraining children for healthcare interventions. However where child health practitioners have specific guidelines for restraining children, this may not be the case in other branches and could lead to conflict and misunderstanding between the nurse and the parents.

The Royal College of Nursing (RCN) Restraining, Holding Still and Containing Children and Young People: Guidance for Nursing Staff, issued in April 2003, states that 'Registered nurses are bound by a duty of care and are accountable for promoting and protecting the rights and best interests of their patients'. Where the use of restraint, holding still and containing children and young people is concerned, nurses must consider the rights of the child and the legal framework surrounding children's rights, including the Human Rights Act (Wadham and Mountfield, 2001), the UN Conventions on the Rights of the Child (UNICEF, 1989), Consent and Capacity Assessment. The document further clarifies the principles of good practice. Holding a child still for a particular clinical procedure such as the insertion of eye drops, requires the nurse to 'give careful consideration of whether the procedure is really necessary, and whether urgency in an emergency situation prohibits the exploration of alternatives. Anticipate and prevent the need for holding, through giving the child information, encouragement, distraction and if necessary using sedation. In all but the very youngest children obtain the child's consent or assent for any situation which is not a real emergency'. The RCN also states that many nurses do not receive specific training in techniques of restraint and containment, and as a result lack confidence in using these techniques. They recommend that organisations undertake an organisational-wide risk assessment to assess the particular risks in each clinical area that provides treatment for children, thus identifying staff training needs.

THINKING POINT

TAKE A LOOK AT YOUR OWN PRACTICE AREA.

1. Do you provide treatment for children and young people?
2. Do you have a policy and training provision on restraint and holding still?
3. Have you had training in this area?
4. If the answer to question 2 or 3 is no you may find it helpful to obtain a copy of the RCN document and as the RCN recommend, forward this to your risk managers for implementation.

Consent

Consent is seen as a fundamental legal and ethical right for adult patients to determine what happens to their own bodies and is a major component of the Nursing and Midwifery Council (NMC) Code of Standards of Conduct, Performance and Ethics for Nurses and Midwives issued in May 2008. Valid consent to treatment is therefore absolutely central in all forms of healthcare and is seen as a matter of common courtesy between health professionals and their patients. Consent lies at the heart of the relationship between patient and client and is a fundamental part of good practice and a legal requirement (DoH 2001). Any adult of sound mind who is classed as a subject of the law can refuse to accept treatment irrespective of need or catastrophic outcomes. However the issue is not so simple where children are involved, where there is a question of what, if any, consent is required, especially in an emergency. Children in this aspect are classed as 'objects of the law' and therefore do not have the same rights as an adult who is classified as a subject of the law. The legal framework is governed, in the criminal law, by the law of assault and, in the civil field, by the duty to take reasonable care of a patient by the exercise of proper professional competence and to act in the best interest of the patient. Hedley (2002) argues that the real difficulties lie in the areas where consent is being refused by a child whom the clinician believes to have the capacity to consent. This is seen by many medical practitioners and nurses as a grave step to override and, if the refusal to consent is contrary to the best interests of the child, the decision to treat is most likely to be made by the court.

Children with mental health or learning disabilities are another area that causes concern when consent for treatment or intervention is required. The NMC code states that 'you must be aware of the legislation regarding mental capacity, ensuring that people who lack capacity remain at the centre of decision making and are fully safeguarded'. However, it must never be assumed that children with mental health or learning disabilities are not competent to make their own decisions; many of these children, if given the information in an appropriate way and well supported through the decision-making process will be deemed to be competent to consent to any intervention or treatment offered.

Gone are the days when doctors adopted the paternalistic attitude that 'doctor knows best'. It is almost universally accepted that the doctrine of 'informed patient consent' is the present position. Informed consent when correctly obtained reminds the health practitioner to respect patient's autonomy and their right to bring personal values into making healthcare decisions that affect them (Cooke, 2005). This concept involves four elements, the provision of information, assessment of the patient's understanding and their capacity to make decisions and the freedom to choose. Informed consent works well when dealing with a competent adult but what about the pre-verbal child? There is a general belief that parents or legal guardians have the authority or the right to give consent by 'proxy' and in practice this is widely accepted. However, informed consent involves personal judgements about the treatment or the intervention which is based on personal beliefs, values and goals. This cannot be directly determined where the pre-verbal child is concerned. It is assumed by many professionals that the parents have the best interest of their child at heart and aim to seek the best health care available for them. However in agreeing to a course of action involving their child they cannot be assumed to know for certain what their pre-verbal child would consent to were he or she able to give informed permission to any intervention. The best interest philosophy can be difficult to define with the many social, religious, philosophical and cultural ideas about what constitutes acceptable child rearing and welfare in today's multicultural society. When babies and young children are being cared for it is not always practicable to seek parents' consent on every occasion for every routine intervention such as blood or urine tests or even X-rays. However in the eyes of the law obtaining written consent is a legal requirement. When children are admitted it is good practice to discuss with the parents what routine procedures will be necessary and obtain their consent for the interventions in advance. When obtaining consent from parents it is essential that you identify who has the parental responsibility, as they are the people entitled to give consent on behalf of the child. Not all parents have responsibility, for example unmarried fathers do not automatically have such responsibility although they can acquire it through marriage or recourse to the law. The safest route in these situations is to get the mother to sign and agree on any treatment, as mothers who have given birth to a child nearly always have the responsibility for that child.

Obtaining consent from children and young people may be 'second nature' within paediatric units where the staff are well aware of the issues and the law surrounding children; however this understanding may not be the same in other areas where child care is provided. If your work involves the provision of health care for children there is a need to make sure firstly that you know the law, secondly that you are able to demonstrate that you have acted in their best interest and thirdly that you have consent to do what you propose to do.

Retinopathy of prematurity

Retinopathy of prematurity

Many problems such as those with a genetic, or inherited component begin before birth; however the treatment required may well persist until old age. This is in fact the patient's journey from cradle to grave. This journey is far from being seamless and can cause problems for patients, families and the practitioner dealing with the issues. The transition from child to adult is not always as smooth and friction free as it could be but good interagency communication helps to make the transition painless.

One area of growth is the provision of neonatal care with many very premature and very low birth weight infants now surviving. This is not without its problems; many of these infants are now surviving with varying degrees of retinopathy of prematurity (ROP), from mild sight defects to complete blindness. Advancements in screening and technology for treatment have resulted in more of these very preterm infants surviving but with the numbers of babies identified with ROP rising. The British Paediatric and Ophthalmic Association in 1995 (RCO and BAPM, 1995) estimated the incidence varies between 30% and 60% in babies weighing less than 1500g and less than 31 weeks gestation. ROP is a major cause of blindness in children in developed countries. However it is a treatable disease with a decline in the incidence in the older premature infant, but with a rise in the very low birth weight infant. The challenge to any neonatal practitioner is to prevent it happening in the first place. There are now monitors which measure oxygen in the blood stream by the arterial route or oxygen saturation of tissues. What is missing is a definitive guide to identify what the optimal level of oxygen should be to prevent ROP. When a very preterm infant is admitted to a neonatal intensive care unit the emphasis is placed on maintaining respiratory and cardiac functions. It is of little benefit to have a child with good eyesight but unable to breathe; this may be seen as a cynical point of view, but the first area that parents always inquire about is their infant's breathing, and the amount of oxygen they are receiving. When an infant is diagnosed with ROP the challenge for the nursing staff begins. How do you explain to parents that their child has a sight problem and still maintain the parent's ability to 'bond' with their baby?

It is now more than 50 years since the association of oxygen therapy and ROP was first described and there is still no definitive evidence on which to base policy. Neonatologists vary widely in their opinions and practices regarding oxygen management in both the early and later neonatal courses of preterm infants. There is a variety of oxygen saturations, those who favour the lower range of less than 90% favour the evidence that higher saturation of partial oxygen (SpO2) and higher partial arterial oxygen (PaO2) levels may contribute to increased incidence of severe ROP, chronic lung disease and brain damage due to oxidative injury (Cole, 2004). However, recent findings have raised concern with these practitioners who practice with the lower ranges of oxygen saturations of below 90%. While they are associated with less ophthalmic and pulmonary problems, these restrictive oxygen limits may be involved in increased incidences of patent ductus arteriosus, pulmonary vascular resistance, apnoea and bradycardia that may be compromising the survival and neurological development outcomes.

All infants with stage 3 disease and those who have been treated should be reviewed in the pre-school years to monitor the development of vision, refractive status and ocular motility as the incidence of strabismus is raised from 6% to over 30%. Myopia is a well known complication of ROP and long-term complications include the risk of developing retinal detachment, which may occur at any time of life (Cole, 2004).

The dilemma of providing care does not stop with the completion of neonatal care, as the children with ROP who survive are then discharged home and into paediatric ophthalmic services. To the parents this is new territory and they are faced with new practitioners whose speciality may not be primarily concerned with children and who may not be aware of the trials and tribulations that have gone before. Many of these parents demonstrate their anxieties by comparing the two areas; comments are made such as 'they did not do that on the neonatal unit', or 'I have not been shown that way before'. They compare the care givers and the care that is given often in uncomplimentary ways, which has the effect of causing friction between the parents and the care givers, often leading to misunderstandings.

Where does this leave the practitioner providing the care for the infants? How can they provide evidence-based care and operate with the best interest of the child when there is no definitive evidence on which to base their care? There is a great risk of litigation under the category of torts, a civil wrong in which a person has breached a legal duty with subsequent harm caused to another. This breach of duty can be either intentional or negligent and results in defined roles of the injured party and the person accused of the wrong doing. Children, unlike adults, have the law behind them and this gives them the right until they reach their eighteenth birthday to sue for injuries suffered during their childhood. This further adds to the risk for the practitioners, and any documentation needs to be written in a clear and concise manner, be dated and timed and have a very clear signature for any incident that occurs, as this may be required in eighteen years time to prove evidence of the care given and that the duty of care had not been breached. There is also a need to clearly document who gave consent and what kind of consent was given, oral, either face to face or over the telephone, implied or no consent given or not required (NMC, 2001). Without this written document, how could you provide evidence of implied consent in eighteen years time? Many practitioners still consider this area as a 'chore' but where the law is concerned, if it is not written in black and white, it has not been done. The lack of written evidence is often the area that causes great concern to the legal profession and health practitioners who are called to give evidence in court cases for neglect of duty of care to children.

National Service Framework for Children 2004

National Service Framework

At the heart of the Children's National Service Framework (DES, 2004) is a fundamental change in thinking about health and social care services. It is intended to lead to a cultural shift, resulting in services which are designed and delivered around the needs of children and families using the services, not around the needs of organisations. This Framework adds another dilemma for practitioners as the recommendations require a totally different mindset that not only requires an increase in staffing levels in both health and social services, but the ability to work in a coordinated set up, to improve access to services for all children according to their needs and to tackle health inequalities.

Part I of the framework sets out five standards which are designed to help the National Health Service, Local Authority and their partner agencies achieve a high quality service provision for all children and young people and their parents or carers.

The five standards are:

Standard 1 The health and well-being of all children and young people is promoted and delivered through a coordinated programme of action, including prevention and early intervention wherever possible to ensure long-term gain, led by the NHS in partnership with local authorities. The emphasis here is on the child Health Promotion Programme, which aims to promote the health and well-being of children and help to reduce health inequalities. It addresses the needs of children from pre-conception to adulthood and integrates pre-school and school age health promotion and assessment including screening and immunisation, which is delivered by a range of health and social care practitioners working together to provide a comprehensive family support services. However this relies on the different agencies working to the same agenda and providing a comprehensive training scheme for the many practitioners involved in providing this standard of care. The central theme is the importance of assessing the needs of children and young people and intervening early, which is not without its problems, as the ability to assess the needs and provide the intervention requires a good knowledge of child development and family functions. This knowledge and understanding would be readily available in specific child health organisations but could the same be said for other agencies that are providing care for children and young people?

Standard 2 Parents and carers are enabled to receive the information, services and support which will help them to care for their children and equip them with the skills they need to ensure that their children have optimum life chances and are healthy and safe. The emphasis is placed on the importance of providing up-to-date information and education for parents which includes how to manage their child's illness and any problems that may occur. Part of this information is highlighting the range of services available to provide further support. When dealing with children this standard identifies the need for parents with specific needs such as relationship conflict, mental health problems, addiction to alcohol and drugs, teenage parents or parents of disabled children to have their needs identified early and to be provided with effective multi-agency support. This implies that practitioners dealing with children need to keep themselves up-to-date with research, not only within their specialist field but also research and development about children. The practitioner needs to understand how the parents' lifestyle could be impacting on the child and their compliance to the treatment offered and have a working knowledge of what services are available and how to refer these cases. In order for this to be effective, services need to be available and coordinated across child and adult services so that the support for parents is available and to ensure the children's safety.

Standard 3 Children and young people and families receive high quality services which are coordinated around their individual and family needs and take account of their views. This standard is applied to staff, who work with children and young people across agencies and are required to develop a common core of skills, knowledge and competencies. Staff training and development programmes should ensure safe practice and comply with clinical governance and good practice guidance. Health services and local authorities should have in place systems to deliver continuous improving high quality child-centred services. This would rely on a more systematic approach being taken to improve access to services in order to ensure that children get the services that they need. Added to this is the need for areas that provide care for children to be staffed by appropriately qualified child health practitioners and not just the token child health practitioner being appointed to try and meet the requirements.

Standard 4 All young people have access to age-appropriate services which are responsive to specific needs as they grow into adulthood. Services need to support young people to achieve their full potential by providing targeted support through coordinated working, and improved access especially when addressing the needs of disabled young people, young people in special circumstances and those who live in rural areas. This is especially a difficult area when transition to adult services is involved. This needs to be planned and coordinated around the needs of each young person to maximise their health outcomes, their life chance opportunities and their ability to live independently, especially where ophthalmic issues are concerned, as they are likely to be long-term and may be complex conditions which need extended care.

Standard 5 All agencies work to prevent children suffering harm and to promote their welfare, provide them with the services they require to address their identified needs and safeguard children who are being or who are likely to be harmed. Safeguarding and promoting the welfare of children is to be a priority to all agencies working in partnership to plan and provide coordinated and comprehensive services in line with national guidance and legislation. This requires an up-to-date profile of the local population to be compiled to facilitate the identification and assessment of children and young people who may be vulnerable and require services. This would also require a range of high quality and integrated services to be available to meet these assessed needs of the child and young person who has been, or is at risk of being, harmed, abused or neglected. Added to this there is also the need for effective supervision to be provided to all staff who work with children to ensure high quality services and that clear accurate, comprehensive and contemporaneous records are kept.

Full implementation of the standards is expected to take up to ten years though the pace of change and the immediate local priorities may vary. However change can be stressful and can be a frightening experience to some, especially where assessment on the quality of services is part of the implementation. Lack of staff and recruitment and retention play a big part in the development of the framework which will only succeed if staff at all levels seize the opportunities provided by the National Health Service Framework for Children and Young People.

Protecting the vulnerable child

Protecting the vulnerable child

Child abuse and neglect are generic terms encompassing all ill-treatment of children including serious physical and sexual assaults as well as cases where the standard of care does not adequately support the child's health or development. Children can be abused or neglected through the infliction of harm or through the failure to act to prevent harm. Abuse can occur in a family or an institutional or community setting, such as a hospital or clinic. Significantly, a child can sustain ocular trauma and other conditions due to various types of abuse, such as physical abuse, sexual abuse and neglect.

Children who are defined as being 'in need', under the Children Act 1989, are those whose vulnerability is such that they are unlikely to reach or maintain a satisfactory level of health development, or their health and development will be significantly impaired without the provision of services (s17 (10) of the Children Act 1989). The critical factors to be taken into account in deciding whether a child is in need under the Children Act 1989 are what will happen to a child's health or development without services, and the likely effect the services will have on the child's standard of health and development. Some children may be considered as being in need because they are suffering or are likely to suffer significant harm. This is the threshold that justifies compulsory intervention in the family life in the best interest of children (Children Act 1989).

Following the publication of *Working Together to Safeguard Children* (DoH, 1999), The Framework for the Assessment of Children in Need (DoH, 2000) and the Laming Report in 2003 on the death of Victoria Climbié the issue of child protection became part of everybody's role, and child protection training in the health service became a priority with the publication of *What to Do if You're Worried a Child is Being Abused* (DoH, 2003) in 2003. Each hospital trust was given a directive that they had to identify a named doctor and nurse with specific responsibility for child protection and put in place a clear child protection policy. The Department of Health had in the 1999 document revised the four categories of child abuse and enhanced the definitions, making them clearer with the aim of reducing the possibility of ambiguity becoming a problem. However this still leaves the practitioner, when faced with a possible child protection case, to decide what constitutes an accident or a non-accidental injury; even though the definitions have been enhanced it is still not clear cut as to what constitutes a non-accidental injury. The Department of Health has tried to help in this area by distributing to every nurse on the Nursing and Midwifery Council register the What to Do if You're Worried a Child is Being Abused document (DoH, 2003). This document gives clear guidance on what to do, who to report to, what will happen following referral and what further contributions may be required.

Working Together to Safeguard Children (DoH, 1999) sets out definitions and examples of what constitutes abuse in four categories:

- physical abuse
- emotional abuse
- sexual abuse
- neglect.

Physical abuse may involve hitting, shaking, throwing, poisoning, burning or scalding, drowning, suffocating or otherwise causing physical harm to a child. Physical harm may also be caused when a parent or carer feigns the symptoms of, or deliberately causes ill health to a child they are looking after. This situation is commonly described using terms such as factitious illness by proxy. Damage to eye orbits and penetrative eye injuries such as a simple 'black eye' could be classified as an accidental injury (AI) or non-accidental injury (NAI). There are also issues around the identification of NAI in the Ophthalmic Emergency and Accident department. A child who presents with a displaced retina or petechial haemorrhage of the eye could have been a victim of hitting, shaking or throwing, but these signs could also occur due to an accident. In order to distinguish between the two injuries and be able to make an informed decision, practitioners need to obtain a full comprehensive history from both the child and the parents. It is the history and the coherence of the accounts of what happened that make the difference between an accident and a non-accidental injury. However one area of this category that is causing a lot of problems is 'hitting' a child by a parent. English law unlike Scotland and Southern Ireland has declined to instigate a total ban on this practice. The English law has allowed parents to use reasonable chastisement on their own child, without leaving a mark and without the aid of an implement. Should a mark be left this is classed as physical abuse. Practitioners need to be aware of this anomaly in the law and be able to act accordingly. However should a parent be observed chastising a child, there is a need to decide if the chastisement being used is 'reasonable' or has an implement been used, which would indicate that a battery has been committed; if so the appropriate action needs to be taken to protect the child from physical abuse. However, many practitioners shy away from this aspect and fail to probe and ask the difficult questions, mainly because they are unsure of what to do if the answer suggests non-accidental injury.

Emotional abuse is the persistent emotional ill treatment of a child so as to cause severe and persistent adverse effects on the child's emotional development. It may involve conveying to children that they are worthless or unloved, inadequate, or valued only insofar as they meet the need of another person. It may feature age or developmentally inappropriate expectations being imposed on children. It may involve causing children frequently to feel frightened or in danger, or the exploitation or corruption of children. Some level of emotional abuse is involved in all types of ill treatment of a child, though it may occur alone. Identification of this type of abuse is difficult and may not be obvious until late into teenage years or later. This may manifest itself in children being uncooperative and non-compliant, especially when diagnosed with a sight problem and being prescribed 'glasses'. The practitioner may overhear the parent or carer making remarks about the child being 'ugly' with those things on their face. The child may present as being withdrawn, very quiet, or have a frightened look. These need to be identified and reported as they may not be due to the child's fear of the unknown such as the hospital setting, but the more sinister aspect of child abuse.

Sexual abuse involves forcing or enticing a child or young person to take part in sexual activities, whether or not the child is aware of what is happening. The activities may involve physical contact, including penetrative or non-penetrative acts. They may include non-contact activities, such as involving children in looking at, or in the production of, pornographic material or watching sexual activities, or encouraging children to behave in sexually inappropriate ways. This definition may be difficult to identify in ophthalmic practice, but practitioners need to look at eye infections and think 'how did this occur', 'how did this child get this infection' especially where there is evidence of infection through sexually transmitted diseases in any eye swabs taken. Is the explanation offered by the parents/carer coherent, plausible and consistent? Does it match the timing, site and spread of the injury? Is it compatible with the child age and mobility? Most important, if the child can explain coherently, what is his/her account of how the infection occurred?

Neglect is the persistent failure to meet a child's basic physical and/or psychological needs, likely to result in the serious impairment of the child's health or development. It may involve a parent or carer failing to provide adequate food, shelter and clothing, failing to protect a child from physical harm or danger, or the failure to ensure access to appropriate medical care or treatment. It may also include neglect of, or unresponsiveness to a child's basic emotional needs. This category is usually identified by observation of the child and parent interaction, but practitioners need to be aware that all neglect is not malicious. If a child is poorly dressed, but appears to be growing and well fed, it may be that the parents have a limited income and are spending the money on feeding the child. However help may be needed as these children could be classed as children in need under section 17 of the Children Act 1989, but not necessarily suffering significant harm under section 31 of the Children Act 1989. However they still need to be referred to Social Services for help to prevent any further decline in their development. Neglect could also be identified in a case of the parent(s) not complying with the administration of eye drops, or failing to attend follow up clinics. This type of neglect would however be seen as true neglect and the child in this case could be seen to be in danger of significant harm, without the prescribed treatment being administered correctly. Again these cases do need to be referred to Social Services for help and guidance.

Handling disclosure information about child abuse

Handling disclosure information

Having talked about protecting the vulnerable child and looked at the categories, the reader is probably asking the question 'how do we handle a disclosure?' This information may come from a child, teenager or even an adult. However the guidelines are exactly the same. There is no time limit on a person disclosing child abuse and the information is treated in the same way regardless of the age of the person.

If a child/young person/adult disclosed to you that they have been abused:

● Stay calm and listen to what is being said.

- Take what is being said seriously, regardless of the age of the person.

- Reassure the child/young person/adult, but do not agree to keep the information secret.

- Allow the claimant to talk about the situation but do not pressurise them for more information.

- Try to get another person to listen to the disclosure; this is good practice as the child/young person/adult may deny the conversation, if they still feel threatened by the abuser.

- Report the incident; if appropriate remain with the child/young person/adult; discuss the situation with a senior manager/member of staff.

- Follow your local policy and procedure; make sure that the conversation is recorded in a written format. The written report needs to identify exactly what has been said to you, not what you thought had been said. Write the report clearly and factually and if appropriate get the child/young person/adult to read what you have written and sign it. This provides further evidence and is seen as good practice by the legal profession.

- Report to Social Services usually by telephone and follow this up in writing within 48 hours.

- Social Services acknowledge receipt of the referral and decide on the action taken, within one working day.

THINKING POINT

TAKE A FEW MINUTES TO READ THROUGH THIS SCENARIO FROM PRACTICE AND REFLECT ON HOW YOU WOULD RECORD THE PARENT'S VISITS AND THEIR ACTIONS AND THE SUPPORT YOU COULD OFFER FOR THIS FAMILY:

Baby A, who is now approximately 12 weeks old and had been born very premature, was diagnosed with a sight problem related to ROP. He was prescribed glasses to assist with his overall growth, and development of his visual acuity.

continued overleaf

It was obvious to the nursing staff that the glasses were helping as they recorded in the care plan that when he wore the glasses he was alert and looking around, focusing on faces when picked up. When the glasses were removed he tended to lie in his cot and was not interested in his surroundings.

To see a baby in a neonatal unit with 'glasses' was 'strange' and other parents soon began to comment on the baby's appearance. This had an adverse effect on the parents who, when visiting, their first action was to remove the spectacles, as they did not wish their child to be seen as a 'freak'.

The nursing staff faced a daily challenge from these parents and their non-compliance in the treatment prescribed for their child. The Children Act 1989 requires parents and professionals to abide by the principle of what is 'in the best interest of the child'. In this incident the nurses providing care were looking at this principle, but what about the parents?

Conclusion

This chapter has identified the significant current ethical and legal issues related to ophthalmic paediatric practice that clearly provide major challenges for practitioners in the future. The impact of changes in the diagnosis, treatment and delivery of paediatric care is now being seen across all areas, whether it be in health or social care. The expansion of the National Health Service and private provision has resulted in more children being identified as requiring ophthalmic treatment which as described in the chapter, is not without its challenges and dilemmas. The impact of the age changes to 19 and 25 years as cited in the Children Act 2004 will have a huge impact on the future planning requirements for the provision of facilities for children's services. The implementation of the NHS frameworks will impart a fundamental change in thinking about health and social care services, hopefully leading to a cultural shift around the delivery of services, therefore producing a seamless service which allows transferral from child to adult services, making it as painless as it can be for the child, family, and/or carers. Many of the ophthalmic problems that occur in children are life-long issues and this area is clearly a 'cradle to the grave' requirement for care. In order to support these children through the changes, practitioners in all areas now need a sound professional knowledge and understanding of child development and the law surrounding children in order to deliver the very best evidence-based practice. Many of these issues, such as best practice, professional accountability and professional knowledge, will be reinforced in Chapter 9, with particular reference to older people, and Chapter 10, which examines evidence-based ophthalmic practice. It is hoped however that at the completion of this chapter the reader's knowledge and understanding of the important ethical and legal issues that surround care-giving to children and young adults has increased and will now form the basis for a broader outlook on their ophthalmic practice areas.

References

Children Act (1989). *Children Act* London: HMSO Publications.

Children Act (2004). *Children Act* London: HMSO Publications.

Cole, Cynthia H. (2004). 'Scientific uncertainty, randomized trials, and resolution of neonatal oxygenation dilemma.' *Neonatal Intensive Care* 17 (4): 16—18.

Cooke, Richard W.I. (2005). 'Good practice in consent.' *Seminars in Fetal and Neonatal Medicine* 10 (63): 71.

Department for Education and Skills (2004). *National Service Framework for Children, Young People and Maternity Services*. London: Department for Education and Skills.

Department of Health (1999). *Working Together to Safeguard Children: A guide to the inter-agency working to safeguard and promote the welfare of children.* London: The Stationery Office.

Department of Health (2000). *Framework for Assessment of Children in Need.* London: The Stationery Office.

Department of Health (2001). *Good practice in consent implementation guide. Consent to examination or treatment*. London: Department of Health Publications

Department of Health (2003). *What to Do If You're Worried a Child is Being Abused.* London: Department of Health.

Hedley, M. (2002). 'Treating children: whose consent counts?' *Current Paediatrics* 12: 463—4.

Laming, Lord (2003). *The Victoria Climbie Inquiry.* London: HMSO.

Nursing and Midwifery Council (2001). *Guidelines on Record Keeping.* London: Department of Health.

Nursing and Midwifery Council (2008). *The Code, Standards of Conduct, Performance and Ethics for Nurses and Midwives.* London: Department of Health.

Royal College of Nursing (2003). *Restraining and Holding Still and Containing Children and Young People: Guidance for Nursing Staff.* London: RCN.

Royal College of Ophthalmologists & British Association of Perinatal Medicine (1995). *Retinopathy of Prematurity Guidelines for Screening and Treatment. The report of a Joint Working Party.* London: RCOP.

UNICEF (1989). *The United Nations Convention on the Rights of the Child.* London: Stationery Office.

Wadham, John, and Mountfield, Helen (2001). *Human Rights Act 1998* 2nd ed. London: Blackstone Press Ltd.

Chapter 9
Older people and ophthalmic practice
Susan Watkinson and Paul Buka

Visual impairment and demographic changes

National Service Frameworks and government policy

Older people and common eye conditions

Physical and psychosocial aspects of visual impairment in older people

Partnership for promoting health

Introduction

In the preceding chapter the 'cradle to grave' concept was highlighted as a requirement for the delivery of ophthalmic care. Clearly, some of the ophthalmic conditions occurring in childhood, such as congenital cataract, congenital glaucoma, refractive error and retinopathy of prematurity will require life-long management. In contrast, however, there are ophthalmic conditions giving rise to visual impairment which arise solely as a result of the ageing process. Thus, the aim of this chapter is to discuss some of the current issues and future challenges posed by older people who, because of the ageing process, develop such sight-threatening conditions.

Undoubtedly, with the predicted growth in the UK's older population, the main ocular conditions such as age-related macular degeneration (AMD), primary open-angle glaucoma (POAG), diabetic retinopathy, and refractive errors will give rise to an increase in visual impairment. Again, it is important to reiterate that demographic change remains a major challenge for the future. Alongside demographic change other significant challenges will include implementing government policy, reaching key targets identified within National Service Frameworks, and addressing the physical and psychosocial implications of visual impairment.

The need for ophthalmic practitioners to meet the continuing challenges of their role as health educators in promoting long-term health and delivering evidence-based care to improve eye health screening and low vision services will also be discussed. Older people need relevant information, help and support to gain sufficient control over the management of their visual problems. Self-management can help to promote and maintain self-esteem and confidence. In turn, this facilitates decision-making about appropriate lifestyle changes to maintain ocular health and re-establish a longer-term quality of life.

Finally, ophthalmic practitioners need to promote their role as the older person's advocate in future policy-making for more effective resources. Economically, for the future, it will be more cost-effective to prevent, or reduce visual impairment, thus resulting in more independence and a longer-term quality of vision and lifestyle for the older person.

Visual impairment and demographic changes

Demographic changes

Globally, in 2002 more than 161 million people were visually impaired, of whom 124 million people had low vision and 37 million were blind (WHO, 2004). By age, more than 82% of all people who are blind are 50 years of age and older, and represent 19% of the world's population. Geographically, more than 90% of the world's visually impaired live in developing countries. By gender, women are at greater risk of vision loss and nearly 82% of those with visual impairment are above the age of 50 years (WHO, 2004).

In the United Kingdom, demographic changes have resulted in a steadily increasing ageing population. It is estimated that by 2025 one-fifth of the UK population (12.8 million people) will be over the age of 65. The number of people aged 80 and older, however, will grow fastest and reach 3.5 million by the year 2025 (Department of Health (DoH), 2001a). In the UK, sight-loss is largely an age-related phenomenon and 70% of all people with sight problems are aged 65 and over (DoH, 2001a). With such a predicted growth, an age-related incidence of visual impairment will also increase. Serious sight problems are also likely to be experienced by people in the 80 and over age group.

Demographic changes will undoubtedly impact financially on the healthcare services in the future management and care of older people with visual impairment. The National Health Service (NHS) and local authorities currently spend almost £20 billion annually on long-term and residential care and nursing homes to support older people with visual impairment (DoH, 2001a). For the future, helping such people to maintain independence in their own homes would be much more cost-effective and would also reduce the burden of failing sight on the health services for the future.

National Service Frameworks and government policy

National Service Frameworks

The National Service Frameworks (NSFs) will present practitioners with the major challenge of trying to meet the targets set for improving standards in the delivery of high quality healthcare services for the future. The most significant NSFs related to older people are:

- The NSF for Older People (DoH, 2001a)
- The NSF for Diabetes: standards (DoH, 2001b)
- The NSF for Diabetes: Delivery Strategy (DoH, 2003)
- Improving Diabetes Services – The NSF Two Years On (DoH, 2005a).

The NSF for Older People (DoH, 2001a)

This framework has been established to look at the problems facing older people receiving care in order to deliver higher quality services (DoH, 2001a). It is underpinned by eight key standards, of which Standard 6 relates to the number of falls in older people. The aim here is to reduce the number of falls that result in serious injury and ensure effective treatment and rehabilitation for those who have fallen (DoH, 2001a). Falls are a major cause of disability and the leading cause of mortality resulting from injury in people aged over 75 in the UK (NICE, 2004). In

1999, there were 647,721 Accident and Emergency attendances and 204,424 admissions to hospital for fall-related injuries in the UK population aged 60 years or over (NICE, 2004). Major risk factors for falling are diverse, but visual impairment ranks significantly among them. This reinforces the need for regular visual assessment (NICE, 2004).

Older people living in residential and nursing homes constitute a particularly high-risk group for falls. Research evidence suggests that visual impairment is strongly associated with falls and hip fractures (Abdelhafiz and Austin, 2003; Ivers et al., 2003). Visual impairment, however, is not only caused by loss of visual acuity. Reduced visual field, which also increases with age, impaired contrast sensitivity, and cataract may also influence this association with falls. Annually, the NHS spends £1.7 billion on treating hip fractures resulting from falls that occur mainly in older people whose failing eyesight has often been a contributory factor (DoH, 2001a). Legood et al., (2002) found that older people with eyesight problems are seven times more likely to fall and sustain a serious injury. It is encouraging, however, that the situation could be improved by adding the treatment of poor vision to exercise and hazard management in the home. This has resulted in an additional 14% reduction in the annual fall rate compared with no intervention (Day et al., 2002).

The NSF for Diabetes: standards (DoH, 2001b)

Diabetes is becoming a more common condition world-wide. It can affect people of all ages in every population. Socially disadvantaged groups in affluent societies and people from black and minority ethnic communities (especially those of South Asian, African and African-Caribbean descent) are particularly vulnerable (DoH, 2001b). In the UK, diabetes mellitus constitutes a major health challenge for the 21st century. Equally, this condition is probably the single most important future challenge for practitioners working within the healthcare services, but particularly within ophthalmic practice. There are currently over 2.5 million people with this condition and there are more than half a million people with undiagnosed diabetes (Diabetes UK, 2008). With the predicted growth in the older population the incidence of visual impairment due to ocular complications such as diabetic retinopathy will also increase (Diabetes UK, 2008). Of further significance is that within the older population, the burden of diabetic eye disease will also fall disproportionately on members of minority ethnic groups, and the poor (DoH, 2003).

The NSF for diabetes is a concerted effort to make sure that people with diabetes in the UK receive the same excellent standard of care, wherever they live (DoH, 2001b). Embodied in the NSF are the central values of the NHS Plan and The Expert Patient – that good service is patient-focused and the outcome of genuine partnership between the patient and the provider. The framework includes the standards, rationales, and key interventions needed to raise the standards of diabetes care, together with an analysis of the implications for planning services (DoH, 2001b).

The NSF for Diabetes: Delivery Strategy (DoH, 2001b)

This framework sets out national targets against which local NHS performance on the standards in the NSF for Diabetes can be judged (DoH, 2001b). This strategy has prioritised retinopathy screening in the UK as one of two critical national targets. By 2006, a minimum of 80 per cent of people with diabetes should be offered screening for the early detection, and, if needed, treatment of diabetic retinopathy, rising to 100 per cent by the end of 2007 (DoH, 2001b). However, the Department of Health published its Diabetic Retinopathy Screening Statement in 2008 (DoH, 2008) which indicated that the target to screen 100% of people diagnosed with diabetes for diabetic retinopathy was not met by the end of 2007.

Diabetic retinopathy is the leading cause of blindness in people under the age of 60 in industrialised countries (NICE, 2002). However, early detection of sight-threatening diabetic retinopathy and treatment with laser therapy is effective in preventing visual impairment in those people at risk (DoH, 2003).

Improving diabetes services – The NSF two years on (DoH, 2005a)

This report highlights progress over the two years following the publication of the NSF for Diabetes Delivery Strategy. As previously indicated, the main aim of the Diabetes NSF is to move the patient to the heart of the NHS. It requires a system where the person with diabetes is at the centre of decision-making. The expectation is that healthcare professionals will work in partnership with people with diabetes, jointly designing and delivering individual care to meet individual needs. Furthermore, healthcare professionals are required to provide information and support to enable people to become more responsible for the way they live their lives and the possible impact on their own health. This focus on patient involvement and self-management requires considerable change to the way many services are delivered.

Encouragingly, this report suggests that this approach is producing considerable improvements in the services provided to people with diabetes. Nevertheless, enabling patient involvement, and allowing them to join up with clinicians and managers to redesign services to meet new demands will continue to be major challenges for the future. Practitioners will need to be prepared to develop new skills and ways of working. They will also need to be committed to multi-disciplinary working to address the complex health needs of people with long-term conditions such as diabetes.

Older people and common eye conditions

Older people and eye conditions

Common eye conditions arising in older people include age-related macular degeneration (AMD), diabetic retinopathy, cataract, glaucoma, and refractive error. Collectively, these conditions constitute major future challenges for ophthalmic practitioners, such as effective health education and the delivery of high-quality evidence-based care. Current and projected health service reforms will remain heavily committed to preventative regimes of care delivery (Whitehead, 2001). Evidence continues to suggest that practitioners have been, and continue to be, ineffective and inconsistent health education practitioners (Whitehead, 2001). The key aim for the future therefore is to make health education a familiar and recognised part of evidence-based ophthalmic practice to help prevent, or reduce visual impairment to promote longer-term quality of lifestyle and independence.

Age-related macular degeneration

Age-related macular degeneration (AMD) is the most common cause of adult blind registration in many developed countries

(Owen *et al.*, 2003). In the UK, it is the leading cause of visual impairment in people over the age of 65. Owen *et al.* (2003) estimate that there are currently 214, 000 people in the UK with visual impairment caused by this condition. This number is expected to increase to 239,000 by the year 2011.

AMD is an ocular ageing process that takes place in the macula, an area normally responsible for clear and detailed central vision (Kanski, 2007). It is classified as 'Dry' (atrophic) or 'Wet' (neovascular) AMD (NICE, 2008b) 'Dry' AMD is the most common form, usually with an insidious onset and rate of progression (Kanski, 2007). It accounts for approximately 85% of those affected and leads to a mild to moderate loss of sight, although peripheral vision is retained (Kanski, 2007). Currently, no treatment is available for this condition (NICE, 2008b). Although 'Wet' AMD is less common, there are approximately 26,000 new cases in the UK each year (NICE, 2008b). As a condition, it is more devastating because it can lead to severe sight loss within months (Kanski, 2007). It results in blurred and distorted central vision, but some peripheral vision is always retained (Kanski, 2007). Treatment includes photodynamic therapy (PDT), the outcome of which has enabled older people to retain sight and live independently.

Ophthalmic practitioners involved in this area of practice have clearly increased their knowledge and skills in the field of visual assessment, pre-treatment preparation, and post-treatment care and management of the older patient receiving this treatment. Whilst PDT has been an invaluable therapy, it has been found not to be suitable for all types of lesions. The advent of anti-VEGF therapy, administered by an intravitreal technique, has begun to revolutionise the treatment of 'Wet' AMD (Chong, 2006). Inevitably, the current issue surrounding the use of anti-VEGF drugs is one of cost-effectiveness. This is also likely to remain a significant future challenge for the government, ophthalmologists, and ophthalmic practitioners as the UK enters into recession and the prospect of economic downturn and uncertainty for the foreseeable future.

The future challenges for ophthalmic practitioners involved in the delivery of these treatments will undoubtedly be the provision of effective care and management to help their clients come to terms with the visual implications of this condition. Psychological support and counselling skills are essential to help clients overcome the shock of visual loss, provide the basis for their subsequent empowerment and restore sufficient independence to maintain vision and re-establish a good quality of life (Watkinson and Scott, 2007). A further challenge will be the effective delivery of health education underpinned by evidence-based information (Watkinson and Scott, 2007). Giving significant information about AMD empowers the client and meets legal requirements (NMC, 2008).

Although the exact aetiology of AMD is unknown, several risk factors are recognised of which age is the strongest (Chopdar *et al.*, 2003). The vast majority of AMD occurs in people over the age of 50 years and the condition affects more women than men (NICE, 2008b). Other risk factors include smoking, elevated cholesterol, hypertension, cardiovascular disease, race (Caucasians are more likely to have choroidal neovascularisation (CNV)), and family history (AREDS Research Group, 2000).

The most commonly cited risk factor is cigarette smoking; the risk of developing AMD is 3.6 times greater for current and former smokers than for people who have never smoked (NICE, 2008b). Diet and nutrition may also play an important role in AMD. However, evidence from a recent systematic review and meta-analysis indicates that vitamins A, C, E, zinc, lutein, zeaxanthin, (alpha) carotene, (beta) carotene, cryptoxanthin, and lycopene have little or no effect in the primary prevention of early AMD (Chong *et al.*, 2007). Excessive sun exposure has been proposed as a risk factor, but not supported by published studies (Khan *et al.*, 2006).

Undoubtedly, an older person's quality of life declines as a result of the binocular visual loss associated with AMD. This can result in difficulties with daily living, and inability to care for self and dependents. Advice therefore for overcoming the practical problems of daily living, especially reading and writing, and enhancing visual rehabilitation is important. Older people can be referred to the low vision aids clinic, the visually impaired team, social services and the rehabilitation team. Advice can be given about magnifying devices and large print materials to assist with reading. Advice should be given about the need to visit the optician once every two years for an eye test, since eye tests are free for people over the age of 60. Putting older people in touch with patient support groups such as AMD Alliance and the RNIB is advantageous. The Macular Disease Society also offers essential help and support in meeting a wide range of needs, and setting up patient support groups within hospital eye units (Watkinson and Scott, 2007).

In summary, the major concern is that there is currently no cure for AMD. As this condition is likely to give rise to significant visual impairment resulting in a reduced quality of life and functional independence, the adequate provision of social care becomes a priority.

Diabetic retinopathy

Diabetic retinopathy is a vascular complication of diabetes mellitus in which the retinal capillaries tend to degenerate after a number of years (Kanski, 2007). It is a major cause of blindness in people with diabetes (NICE, 2002). The incidence of diabetic retinopathy is related primarily to duration and occurs in individuals with a long history of poorly controlled diabetes (Kanski, 2007). After 20 years from the onset of this condition, more than 60% of those with type 2 diabetes will have diabetic retinopathy with the presence of maculopathy being the major cause of central visual loss (NICE, 2008a). Those with type 1 diabetes will have some degree of retinopathy within 20 years of diagnosis (NICE, 2008a).

One of the most important challenges for ophthalmic practitioners is the need for health education as a preventative strategy. This will form a significant part of the health education management strategy for patients with diabetes mellitus undergoing retinal screening for the future (Watkinson and Chetram, 2005). Primary and secondary prevention of sight-threatening disease is the aim of diabetic retinopathy care (Walker and Rodgers, 2002). It is also the greatest challenge for ophthalmic practitioners. As part of the retinal screening strategy, health education should include the best available research evidence to empower older patients to make decisions about lifestyle changes and gain control over their condition (Watkinson and Chetram, 2005). This provides the basis for more effective self-management of the condition in the long term.

Older patients and their families require information about diabetic retinopathy and how it relates to their diabetes. Maintaining good blood glucose control, for example, is essential.

Levels of blood glucose are set, depending on the individual's risk of macrovascular and microvascular complications, at or below HbA1c 6.5-7.5% (NICE, 2008a). Maintaining good blood pressure is also important. If eye damage is already present, it is recommended that the blood pressure be maintained at or below 140/80mmHg (NICE, 2008a). Adherence to prescribed anti-hypertensive treatment is vital as diabetic patients with hypertension have a poor visual prognosis (NICE, 2008a). Similarly, concordance with drug therapy to lower serum cholesterol levels is important since elevated levels are associated with an increased severity of retinal hard exudates resulting in decreased visual acuity (NICE, 2008a).

Overall, by addressing the current issues and future challenges surrounding diabetic retinopathy, ophthalmic practitioners will be able to extend the scope of their clinical practice by the delivery of important retinal screening and health education strategies for older people with diabetic retinopathy. Continuous updating of their knowledge of diabetes and diabetic retinopathy alongside development of their technical skills will be the ongoing challenges. The outcome of this will be an evidence-based approach to the delivery of high-quality care. Practitioners will also be making a vitally important contribution to achieving government targets as part of a national healthcare screening programme.

Glaucoma

Glaucoma is classified into several types. POAG is a progressive eye disease with a non-dramatic onset affecting 1–2% of people over the age of 40, and 15% of people over 70 (Kanski, 2007). POAG also accounts for 10% of those people registered as partially sighted (RNIB, 2008b).

Older people are at an increased risk of developing this condition because of elevated intra-ocular pressure (IOP), or ocular hypertension (Kass *et al.*, 2002). Age, cup-disc ratio, and IOP are predictive factors for the development of POAG in individuals with ocular hypertension (Gordon *et al.*, 2002). A reduction in IOP is the main way to prevent major sight loss (Gordon *et al.*, 2002; Kass *et al.*, 2002) and thus concordance with ocular hypotensive treatment is vital. The aim is to prevent a total loss of sight and maintain the older person's independence. Older people with POAG may lose quality of life due to the psychological impact of the diagnosis, visual field loss, side-effects of medication, and the cost of treatment (Gray, 2005). There is no cure for POAG, but concordance with prescribed treatment helps the older person to gain good control over the condition. The safety of older people with POAG can be put at risk due to the difficulties of identifying colours, and judging depth, especially in dimly lit areas, or away from the home environment. This may lead to falls which result in injuries requiring hospitalisation (Vu *et al.*, 2005).

Because the majority of older people with POAG are based in the community, and not admitted to ophthalmic wards, the ophthalmic practitioner's role is to focus on empowering the older person through patient education for self-management and control of the condition (Watkinson, 2005). Health education also extends to relatives, who should be made aware of the need for regular sight tests every 2–3 years since there is an increased familial risk of developing the condition. Eye tests are free for relatives of people with glaucoma (age 40 and over) (RNIB, 2008a).

Refractive errors

Another significant problem for community-based practitioners is low vision due to refractive errors. Because of the shift from hospital to community practice more responsibility will be placed on community practitioners to identify patients with a possible refractive error and give appropriate advice to seek help in correcting it and thus prevent deteriorating vision in the longer term. Indeed, uncorrected refractive error was found to be the most common cause of bilateral visual impairment in all decades of life, rising from 0.5% in 40–49 year olds to 13% among those aged 80 years and above (Weih *et al.*, 2000).

Cataract

Cataract is an opacity of the lens and is an abnormal progressive condition (James *et al.*, 2003). Except for the most developed countries, cataract remains the leading cause of blindness in all regions of the world. Associated with ageing, it is even more significant as a cause of low vision (WHO, 2008). It causes half of the blindness worldwide, but vision can be restored by surgery (Vision 2020, WHO, 2009). Cataract surgery is one of the most cost-effective of all health interventions (Vision 2020, WHO,

2009). Low cost consumables and efficient use of resources have reduced the cost of high-quality cataract surgery. However, cost is still a significant barrier to patient uptake of surgery. Therefore, this is a future challenge for governments and donors to commit to cover the cost for poor patients. In the UK, the government has set a target for cataract surgery that is the equivalent to 3,200 cases per 100,000 people aged 65 and over (DoH, 2000).

Importantly, practitioners are faced with the government's targets to provide high quality patient information and a patient focused service (DoH, 2000). Patients need to be given information about the whole treatment pathway, not just individual steps. For example, a patient with a cataract requiring surgery needs standard information about the nature and treatment of this condition at the beginning of the pathway, and the service offered locally (DoH, 2000). The patient is a full partner in the treatment. Where choices exist about treatment, patients need to be provided with the required information to make these choices. The concept of partnership is also instrumental in achieving concordance with prescribed therapy after surgery. Information about possible ocular complications such as secondary glaucoma, or retinal detachment should be given. If pain in and around the eye, or sudden reduced vision, is experienced, the patient needs to contact the hospital immediately for further treatment.

Physical and psychosocial aspects of visual impairment in older people

Physical and psychosocial aspects

An elderly person with impaired vision is more at risk of falls or physical harm. Literature review by Woolf and Åkesson (2003) found that those with impaired visual acuity, cataracts, glaucoma, and retinal degeneration were at such risk. Prior to any discharge from acute care, new guidelines now require a risk assessment for older people who may have been admitted with a history of falls. Having identified visual impairment as one of the contributory factors for falls, Woolf and Åkesson (2003) suggested a two-pronged approach for managing the problem. This included the requirement for risk assessments as well as measures aimed at improving and maintaining bone density. They should also be offered a home hazard assessment and safety intervention/ modifications by a suitably trained healthcare professional (NICE, 2004). An individual with visual impairment may find in time that they can no longer manage to perform daily activities they were previously accustomed to. Considering that reading is one aspect that most people take for granted, loss of vision may have a substantial and negative impact on their lives. Margrain (2000) found that this applied in the majority of the subjects (67%) of his study, who could not read standard newsprint, with a further 40% of these unable to read large print. The provision of low visual aids made a difference for some, giving them some ability to read. In addition, not only are there implications for loss of or limitation of mobility for those older people who drive, but also they are generally accident prone due to increased risk factors associated with visual impairment, according to research on older drivers with cataracts (Owsley *et al.*, 2001).

If a person is considered as a psychosocial animal, which needs to continue to participate in the society they live in, it is not difficult to see how these aspects could be affected by disability and impairment resulting from visual loss. They may feel embarrassed and prefer withdrawal from social activities resulting in isolation. Consequently an individual who suffers from visual impairment may inevitably become isolated and suffer from depression. Recent findings related to the current situation on how we care for older people in the community reported that around half of older people are generally not excluded from society on any of the dimensions, nevertheless:

- 29% are excluded on one dimension
- 13% on two dimensions
- 7% on three or more dimensions…

(Social Exclusion Unit, 2006, p. 7)

Additionally, the social implications for loss of vision may impact on social relationships with caring family members or friends who may themselves be in need of care. It is estimated that the largest group of carers is aged 45–64 years (Donaldson and Donaldson, 2003). In addition to the existing right of the patient to be assessed in the community under section 47 of the NHS and Community Care Act 1990, the Carers Recognition Act 1995 now also requires assessment to include the needs of the carer.

Furthermore a Scottish study by Cox *et al.* (2005) concluded that a significant number of elderly patients with fractured neck of femur representing 239 of 518 patients from the study (46%), suffered from bilateral visual impairment (binocular visual acuity worse than 6/12) and most importantly that a high proportion of this group lived in socially deprived environments (26%), where they were not able to access ophthalmic services. The nature of chronic conditions may be such that individuals' ability to participate in life is limited due to practical difficulties in mobility and access to services. In addition, local authorities should offer practical support with services to benefit the visually impaired individual (RNIB, 2005). One form of assistance could include, where appropriate, a guide dog, a white 'symbol cane', depending on the severity of the impairment. Other practical supportive measures could be all that is required to make the difference between independent living and being admitted to warden controlled accommodation or residential or nursing home. Should any adjustments to access or the living facilities be required, patients are also entitled to a mandatory disabled facilities grant. They may need to assign a friend or family the authority to manage their financial affairs through a 'power of attorney' or an 'enduring power of attorney' (in the event of loss of their mental capacity).

Through referral by an ophthalmic consultant, a person is registered with social services as severely impaired or as blind on presentation of a consultant Letter of Vision Impairment. This would give them access to needs assessments by council rehabilitation officers and will be entitled to benefits such as a blind person's personal allowance £1610 (in 2005–6), a reduction on television licence, disabled person's railcard. They are also protected by Section 21 of the Disability Discrimination Act 1995. Additional benefits will include Attendance Allowance for those over 65 or a Disability Living Allowance for younger individuals.

Additionally, loss of vision may result in stigmatisation, perceived by the individual or real. This may have a psychological effect resulting in social isolation which may be associated with chronically ill individuals.

Partnership for promoting health

One of the biggest challenges facing the ophthalmic practitioner is how to provide health education as part of ongoing treatment. The implication of a rise in the number of older people with diabetes mellitus has also meant that there is an increase in related eye problems. The traditional paternalistic attitudes towards caring should now be replaced by a working relationship of partnership and a concordance between the ophthalmic nurse (other professionals) and the patient. The Health Belief Model (Hochbaum *et al.*, 1992) is one attempt to explain an individual's response to health education and their perceptions of the threat posed by a health problem, such as loss of vision. It also considers benefits of avoiding a perceived threat, as well as any factors which may influence the decision to act. The public may not always be keen to embrace government health education policy, for example on screening eye conditions. This theory has further been modified to explain the circumstances under which people would take health-protective action:

- if they regard themselves as susceptible to the condition
- if they believe it to have potentially serious consequences
- if they believe that a course of action available to them would be beneficial in reducing either their susceptibility to or the severity of the condition
- if they believe that the anticipated barriers to (or costs of) taking the action are outweighed by its benefits.

(Rosenstock, 1990, pp. 42—3)

Alternatively, Integrated Care Models have their emphasis on encouraging improved partnerships and collaboration to improve efficiency in service provision. This is in keeping with current government policy. If an eye condition is addressed in time, it is possible that through treatment the long-term effects may be contained or limited and thus allow the older person to have a better quality of life. The government now recognised the impact of social exclusion by establishing a social exclusion unit in the Deputy Prime Minister's Office to try to improve the quality of life for people such as older people who are isolated.

The government plans to improve the public service performance of service providers by emergency bed days by 5%

by 2008. Effectively, this should improve outcomes for people with long-term conditions through improved primary and community care (DoH, 2005b).

One of the major implications for practitioners is that an increase in life expectancy will result in a greater number of older people needing a wider range of health services including health promotion, illness prevention and rehabilitation. Discussion so far has sought to emphasise that the future role of the ophthalmic practitioner as an effective health educator and promoter will be crucially important in assisting older people with visual impairment to achieve optimal ocular health, a sense of well-being, and a longer-term quality of life. Practitioners in ophthalmic practice have a responsibility to contribute to the maintenance of ocular health and the prevention of ocular disease. The main challenges in achieving this are the maintenance of their own level of competence fostered by a commitment to continuing professional education, effective planning, and the delivery of high quality evidence-based care.

Conclusion

Significantly, the long-term health and management of older people continues to increase its profile on the political agenda. The government White Paper, 'Our health, Our care, Our say: A new direction for community services' (DoH, 2006, p. 7) aims to invest in services for older people as well as to create an ambitious 'new vision for health and social care and promoting ... more personalised care, greater choice and a wider range of services'. Translated into real terms there are resource implications. Without adequate funding, this latest government political will and initiative to improve and address long-term needs may prove to be little more than a white elephant. The ophthalmic needs of older patients, alongside those with long-term conditions will not have been served. The challenge then remains for practitioners to prepare for the planned further shift in emphasis from acute to community care. The NICE (2004) risk assessment guidelines should serve the patient well. The current situation also provides opportunities for practitioners and their organisations to seize the political moment to influence broader debates on global ageing, the determinants of health and the impact of the social environment. It is economically essential in the long-term that the needs of older people with ophthalmic problems are met. Practitioners need to become more politically proactive in acting as advocates or facilitators in policy-making for more effective allocation of healthcare resources and ensuring that such needs are met. Overall, becoming more proactive in practice is a significant future challenge. As already highlighted, this requires commitment to continuing professional education as a basis for updating professional knowledge and demonstrating professional competence in the delivery of evidence-based ophthalmic care. These ongoing challenges will be discussed in more detail in the next chapter.

References

Abdelhafiz, A., and Austin, C. (2003). 'Visual factors should be assessed in older people presenting with falls or hip fracture.' *Age and Ageing* 32: 26–30.

Age-related Eye Disease Study Research Group (2000). 'Risk factors associated with age-related macular degeneration. A case-control study in the Age-Related Disease Study Report 3.' *Ophthalmology* 107: 2224–32.

Chong, E., Wong, T., Kreis, A., Simpson, J., and Guymer, R. (2007). 'Dietary antioxidants and primary prevention of age-related macular degeneration: systematic review and meta-analysis.' *British Medical Journal* 335 (7623): 755–62.

Chong, V. (2006). 'Eye injection and AMD.' *Digest. Journal of the Macular Disease Society* 65–9.

Chopdar, A., Chakravarthy, U., and Verma, D. (2003). 'Age-related macular degeneration.' *British Medical Journal* 326: 485–8.

Cox, A., Blaikie, A., MacEwen, C.J., Jones, D., Thompson, K., Holding, D., Sharma,T., Miller, S., Dobson, S., and Sanders, R. (2005). 'Visual impairment in elderly patients with hip fracture: causes and associations.' *Eye* 19: 652–6.

Day, L., Filders, B., and Gordon, I. (2002). 'Randomised factorial trial of falls prevention among older people living in their own homes.' *British Medical Journal* 325: 128.

Department of Health (2000). *Action on Cataracts*. London: DoH.

Department of Health (2001a). *National Service Framework for Older People*. London: DoH.

Department of Health (2001b). *National Service Framework for diabetes: standards*. London: DoH.

Department of Health (2003). *National Service Framework for diabetes: Delivery Strategy*. London: DoH.

Department of Health (2005a). *Improving Diabetes Services – The NSF Two Years On*. London: DoH.

Department of Health (2005b). *Supporting People with Long Term Conditions. An NHS and Social Care Model to support local innovation and integration*. London: DoH.

Department of Health (2006). *Pilot issue 1- January*. London. DoH. http://www.dh.gov.uk/socialcarebulletin (last accessed 27.11.08).

Department of Health (2008). *Diabetic Retinopathy Screening Statement*. London: Department of Health.

Diabetes UK (2008). *Guide to Diabetes*. London: Diabetes UK. www.diabetes.org.uk/Guide-to-diabetes (last accessed 20.10.08).

Donaldson, L.J., and Donaldson, R.J. (2003). *Essential Public Health* 2nd ed. Newbury: Petroc Press.

Gordon, M., Beiser, J., Brandt, J., Heuer, D., Higginbotham, E., Johnson, C., Keltner, J., Miller, J., Parrish, R., Wilson, M., and Kass, M. (2002). 'The Ocular Hypertension Treatment Study: baseline factors that predict the onset of primary open-angle glaucoma.' *Archives of Ophthalmology* 120 (6): 714–20.

Gray, E. (2005). 'Understanding the role of the glaucoma specialist nurse.' *Nursing Times* 101 (38): 32–4.

Hochbaum, G.M., Sorenson, J., and Lorig, K. (1992). 'Theory in health education practice.' *Health Education Quarterly* 19 (3): 293–313.

Ivers, R.Q., Cumming, R.G., Mitchell, P., Simpson, J.M., and Peduto, A.J. (2003). 'Visual risk factors for hip fracture in older people.' *Journal of American Geriatric Society* 51 (3) March: 356—63.

James, B., Chew, C., and Bron, A.J. (2003). *Lecture Notes on Ophthalmology*. Ninth edition. Oxford: Blackwell Publishing.

Kanski, J. (2007). *Clinical Ophthalmology*. Oxford: Blackwell Publishing.

Kass, M., Heuer, D., Higginbotham, E., Johnson, C., Keltner, J., Miller, J., Parrish, R., Wilson, M., and Gordon, M. (2002). 'The Ocular Hypertension Treatment Study: a randomised trial determines that topical ocular hypotensive medication delays or prevents the onset of primary open-angle glaucoma.' *Archives of Ophthalmology* 120 (6): 701–13.

Khan, J., Shahid, H., Thurlby, D., Bradley, M., Clayton, D., Moore, A., and Yates, J. (2006). 'Age-related macular degeneration and sun exposure, iris colour, and skin sensitivity to sunlight.' *British Journal of Ophthalmology* 90 (27): 39–40.

Legood, R., Scuffham, P., and Cryer, C. (2002). 'Are we blind to injuries in the visually impaired? A review of the literature.' *Injury Prevention* 8 (2): 155–60. http://archopht.ama-assn.org/cgi/content/abstract/109/2/205 (last accessed 23.04.06)

Margrain, T. (2000). 'Helping blind and partially sighted people to read: the effectiveness of low vision aids.' *British Journal of Ophthalmology* 84: 919–21.

National Institute for Clinical Excellence (2002). *Management of Type 2 Diabetes Retinopathy: Early Management and Screening*. www.nice.org.uk/pdf/diabetesretinopathyguideline.pdf (last accessed: 19 November 2004).

National Institute for Clinical Excellence (2004). *New Guidelines for the NHS on the Assessment and Prevention of Falls in Older People.* http://www.nice.org.uk (last accessed 27.11.08)

National Institute for Clinical Excellence (2008a). *The Management of Type 2 Diabetes. NICE clinical guideline 66.* www.nice.org.uk (last accessed 27.11.08)

National Institute for Clinical Excellence (2008b). *Ranibizumab and Pegaptanib for the Treatment of Age-related Macular Degeneration. NICE technology appraisal guidance 155.* http://www.nice.org.uk/nicemedia/pdf/TA155guidance.pdf (Last accessed 27 November 2008).

Nursing and Midwifery Council (2008). *The Code: Standards of Conduct, Performance and Ethics for Nurses and Midwives.* London: NMC. www.nmc-uk.org (last accessed 27 November 2008).

Owen, C., Donoghue, M., and Rudnicka, A. (2003). 'How big is the burden of visual loss caused by age-related macular degeneration in the United Kingdom?' *British Journal of Ophthalmology* 87 (3): 312–17.

Owsley, C., Stalvey, B., Wells, J., Sloane, M., and McGwin, G. (2001). 'Visual risk factors for crash involvement in older drivers with cataracts.' *Archives of Ophthalmology* 119: 881—7.

Rosenstock, I. M. (1990). 'The health belief model: Explaining health behavior through expectancies.' In K. Glanz, F.M. Lewis, & B.K. Rimer (eds.), *Health Behavior and Health Education Theory Research and Practice* (pp. 39–62). San Francisco, CA: Jossey-Bass Publishers.

Royal National Institute of the Blind (2005) *The Benefits of Registering as blind or partially sighted.* London: RNIB.

Royal National Institute of the Blind (2008a). *Getting an Eye Test.* London: RNIB.

Royal National Institute of the Blind (2008b). *Supporting Blind and Partially Sighted People.* London: RNIB.

Social Exclusion Office. www.cabinetoffice.gov.uk (last accessed 23.04.06.

Vu, H., Keeffe, J., McCarty, C., and Taylor, H. (2005). 'Impact of unilateral and bilateral vision loss on quality of life.' *British Journal of Ophthalmology* 89 (3): 360–3.

Walker, R., and Rodgers, J. (2002). 'Diabetic retinopathy.' *Nursing Standard* 16 (45): 46–52.

Watkinson, S. (2005). 'Visual impairment in older people: the nurse's role.' *Nursing Standard* 19 (17): 45–52.

Watkinson, S., and Chetram, N. (2005). 'A nurse-led approach to diabetic retinal screening.' *Nursing Times* 101 (36): 32–4.

Watkinson, S., and Scott, E. (2007). 'The role of the ophthalmic nurse specialist in enhancing the care of patients undergoing photodynamic therapy.' *Journal of ESONT* 1 (3): 27–35.

Weih, L., Van Newkirk, M., McCarty, C., and Taylor, H. (2000). 'Age-specific causes of bilateral visual impairment.' *Archives of Ophthalmology* 118 (2): 264–9.

Whitehead, D. (2001). 'A social cognitive model for health education/health promotion practice.' *Journal of Advanced Nursing* 36 (3): 417–25.

Woolf, A.D. and Åkesson, K. (2003). 'Preventing fractures in elderly people.' *British Medical Journal* 327: 89—95.

World Health Organisation (2004) *Magnitude and Causes of Visual Impairment.* Geneva: WHO.

World Health Organisation (2005). *State of the World's Sight. Vision 2020: the Right to Sight 1999-2005. Executive Summary.* Geneva: WHO.

WHO (2008). *Prevention of Blindness and Visual Impairment.* Geneva: WHO. Available at: www.who.int/entity/blindness/en/ (last accessed 28 February 2009).

WHO (2009). *Vision 2020. The Right to Sight.* Geneva: WHO. Available at: www.v2020.org/ (last accessed 28 February 2009).

Statutes

Carers' Recognition Act (1995)

Chronically Sick and Disabled Persons Act (1970)

Disability Discrimination Act (1995)

Disabled Persons (Services Consultation and Representation) Act (1986)

National Health Service Act (1948)

National Health Service Act (1977)

NHS and Community Care Act (1990)

Chapter 10
Professional education and evidence-based ophthalmic practice
Susan Watkinson

Professional knowledge development
Critical thinking
Research in ophthalmic practice

Introduction

This chapter establishes the link between professional knowledge and evidence-based ophthalmic practice. It also serves as the linchpin for the various aspects of this speciality, explored in preceding chapters, by discussing the application of continuing professional education as a means for ophthalmic practitioners to increase their knowledge and application of research. Such knowledge serves as a platform for developing skills for critical appraisal and care-related decision-making by utilising this research-based evidence in practice.

Undoubtedly, the most important future challenge for ophthalmic practitioners is to undertake their own research in practice. The development of critical thinking skills and a commitment to reflective practice are essential in contributing to evidence-based ophthalmic practice. Government policies have stressed the need for high quality service provision (DoH, 1998, 2000). This includes the promotion of evidence-based practice, patient-centred care, the proliferation of guidelines and protocols, and the implementation of clinical governance. These goals pose significant challenges. Sound clinical judgement about best available evidence to provide best ophthalmic practice is thus vital. The achievement of future goals rests on a commitment to continuing professional education to help increase research-mindedness, develop critical thinking skills and reflective practice as a basis for developing this expertise in professional judgement.

Professional knowledge development

**Professional
knowledge
development**

The relationship between knowledge and research

Professional knowledge development is a complex process and has a significant influence on the relationship between nurse practitioners' perceptions of knowledge and the utilisation of research in practice (Watkinson, 2001). Importantly, ophthalmic practitioners need to be aware of the different sources of knowledge that make up the evidence-base of clinical practice. Indeed, Higgs and Titchen (2000) describe knowledge as fundamental to reasoning and decision-making and thus central to professional practice. Firstly, however, the concept of 'evidence' will be addressed.

The word 'evidence' is rooted in the concept of experience, relating to what is manifest and obvious (Upshur, 2001). In the context of healthcare, Sackett *et al.* (1997, p. 2) defined evidence-based medicine as 'the conscientious, explicit and judicious use of current best evidence about the care of individual patients'. Underpinning this definition was the common assumption that evidence was research-based with specific reference to the quantitative tradition of research. This debate has since moved on. Evidence is viewed as being much broader than that derived purely from research. Higgs and Jones (2000) suggest that evidence-based practice should be considered to be knowledge derived from a variety of sources that has been tested and found credible.

Eraut (1999) similarly argues that all kinds of knowledge are necessary to professional performance and advances three main kinds of knowledge employed in professional practice. These are propositional knowledge, personal knowledge, and process knowledge. He distinguishes three subcategories of propositional knowledge which are:

1) discipline-based theories and concepts, derived from bodies of coherent systematic knowledge (Wissenschaft)

2) generalisations and practical principles in the applied field of professional action

3) specific propositions about particular cases, decisions and actions.

He defines 'process knowledge' as 'knowing how to conduct the various processes that contribute to professional action. This includes knowing how to access and make good use of propositional knowledge' (Eraut, 1999, p. 107). A personal knowledge base includes notes and memories of cases and problems which have been encountered, reflected upon and theorised to varying extents and with varying significance for current practice (Eraut, 1999, p. 17). Broadly, propositional knowledge is formal, explicit, and derived from research and scholarship. Process and personal knowledge constitute non-propositional knowledge that is informal, implicit and derived primarily through practice. Thus, propositional and non-propositional knowledge translate into the 'knowing that' and 'knowing how' identified in Benner's work (1984, 1999). 'Knowing that' relates to traditional, theoretical knowledge such as knowing that most ophthalmic surgical patients suffer from pre-operative anxiety about their forthcoming surgery. 'Knowing how' relates to practical knowledge such as knowledge about how best to allay this anxiety through pre-operative discussion and patient information giving. However, the nature of the ophthalmic nurse practitioner's knowledge is neither wholly 'knowing that' or 'knowing how', but a combination of both. These two perspectives on knowledge form the basis for clinical judgement.

Benner *et al.* (1999) argue that practitioners must be able to draw upon the best scientific evidence available to make sound clinical judgements. At the same time, they must also develop the skills of reasoning in order to develop the best account of a clinical situation to make the best clinical judgements under circumstances of uncertainty. The latter is an interpretative process (Benner *et al.*, 1999). It is important for ophthalmic and general practitioners to be cognisant of the debate surrounding scientific versus intuitive knowledge since their clinical decision-making is both a scientific and interpretative process. The ongoing challenge for practitioners, however, is to decide whether research evidence should inform that clinical decision-making. This means assessing the suitability of this evidence for utilisation in practice.

The relationship between research and practice

The problems of utilising research in practice have been well documented and the specific factors that act as barriers to research utilisation continue to dominate the literature (Walsh, 1997; Dunn *et al.*, 1998; Parahoo, 2000; Bryar *et al.*, 2003). The most significant difficulties encountered in implementing research relate to insufficient time to access and review research reports, and a lack of authority and support to implement findings. Another significant factor is the complexity of professional knowledge development (Watkinson, 2001). If Benner's (1984) model is taken as a conceptual framework, professional knowledge development may be seen as a developmental learning journey from novice to expert stages. Perceptions of the relationship between knowledge and research-based practice will at any time depend on the stage reached in that journey with reference to the practitioner's levels of knowledge, understanding and experience, and the ability to reflect critically on their experiences of clinical practice. These are the essential components that form the basis for enhanced decision-making about the need for implementing research in practice (Watkinson, 2001).

Gerrish and Clayton's (2004) study confirmed lack of time and perceived authority to change practice as factors identified from earlier research studies. Other findings indicated that organisational information, such as policies and audit reports, was drawn upon more frequently than research reports. Also, nurses were skilled at accessing and reviewing evidence, but were less confident about their ability to change practice. Overall, multiple strategies to facilitate and promote evidence-based practice, and managerial support, facilitation, and a culture receptive to change were essential (Gerrish and Clayton, 2004).

On a positive note, the view that nurses in the United Kingdom do not use research has already been challenged (Lacey, 1994, 1996). In the earlier of the two studies, Lacey (1994) found that nurses demonstrated a positive attitude towards research. She claimed many instances of well-informed nurses questioning their practice and implementing research-based change. However, as a pilot study, based on a sample size of only 20 nurses, the overall reliability and generalisability of the findings are questionable It nevertheless provided a springboard for Lacey's (1996) study which showed that 65% of nurses responding to a 6-month post-registration research course evaluation had in some way implemented proposals for change on the basis of research evidence.

More recently, within the area of ophthalmic nursing research, McLauchlan *et al* (2002) concluded that the nursing care of patients undergoing vitreoretinal surgery had developed as a result of undertaking a three-and-a-half-year action research project. Action research was viewed as an appropriate method of addressing the concerns surrounding the posturing of patients after vitreoretinal surgery.

Continuing professional education

Discussion of such evidence reinforces the need for ophthalmic practitioners to become more research-minded by undertaking post-registration research modules such as skills for critical appraisal and evidence-based practice. Indeed, Hutchinson and Johnston's (2004) study identified inadequate skills in critical appraisal as one of the greatest barriers to research utilisation. Undertaking such a module would help to increase research knowledge and facilitate a questioning approach to ophthalmic practice. Effective reading and critical appraisal skills are deemed essential for being able to explore critically the relationship between knowledge, practice, research and education.

Similarly, ophthalmic practitioners undertaking an evidence-based practice module would develop their ability to identify and critically examine priorities for improving practice, and develop their skills of identifying evidence and critically analysing its nature in practice. The skills of evaluating the feasibility and effectiveness of evidence for changes in practice would also be developed.

If the utilisation of research evidence in ophthalmic practice results in better patient outcomes, the important issues of support for the implementation of research findings, the authority to change practice, time constraints, and the ability to critically appraise research with some conviction need to be addressed. These issues will constitute the greatest challenges for the future.

Critical thinking

The discussion so far has focused on continuing professional education as an essential process for developing reflective skills and the ability to think critically. Accessing post-registration research modules as a means to achieving a BSc, or Master's degree will be challenging for the ophthalmic practitioner, but will undoubtedly result in a better appreciation and understanding of the nature of evidence, particularly research evidence. Importantly, it will also encourage critical thinking, and increase knowledge of research appraisal skills and the ability to identify and critique research studies to assess their suitability for implementation in practice.

The many changes that have taken place within the National Health Service have inevitably given rise to increased anxiety about the management of patient care. The need to reinforce a more critical attitude to practice will constitute one of the biggest challenges for ophthalmic practitioners for the 21st century. Achieving it, however, will empower practitioners to assume authority and control over their clinical practice, and exercise patient advocacy.

Underpinning this need is the assumption that ophthalmic practitioners are cognisant of the nature of critical thinking and how to adopt a more critical stance in practice. However, some questions need to be asked. What does being critical mean? Why is it important for clinical practice? What strategies are available for achieving it?

What does 'being critical' mean?

Facione (2007) suggests that critical thinking is self-regulatory judgement that results in the individual being able to interpret, analyse, evaluate and infer. The individual should also be able to explore evidence, concepts, methods, criteria and the context that underpin that judgement. Critical thinking is important for ophthalmic and general practitioners because it is essential as a tool of inquiry. Ennis (2001) suggests that critical thinking means reasonable and reflective thinking focused on deciding what to believe or do, and such thinking is underpinned by a set of critical dispositions and abilities. These have been summarised by Rolfe *et al.* (2001) from the work of Facione (2007) and Brookfield (1997). An ideal critical thinker is someone who is habitually inquisitive, well-informed, open-minded, honest in facing personal biases, willing to reconsider, clear about issues, and diligent in seeking relevant information (Rolfe *et al.*, 2001). From these definitions, critical thinking can be seen as weighing up all the possibilities for action from the best evidence available and being able to make a considered and rational choice.

Benner *et al.* (1999) suggest that being critical means active thinking in practice. 'Thinking' conveys the innovative and productive nature of a practitioner's active thinking in ongoing clinical situations. Thus, 'thinking-in-action' is defined as the patterns and habits of thought and action that are directly tied to responding to patients and families and the demands of a changing situation, including noticing when clinical assumptions are not being met (Benner *et al.*, 1999, p. 570). It is a process of rapid decision-making underpinned by a tacit knowledge base. Eraut (2000) argues that it is a 'ready-to-use' action knowledge. This means that the practitioner reads a situation rapidly with the help of prior knowledge. There is a rapid linkage of that situational understanding with an immediate course of action, using prior knowledge of what has worked before. Benner *et al.* (1999) also believe that alongside 'thinking-in-action', 'reasoning-in-transition' is important. The latter refers to practical reasoning where a clinician takes account of the gains and losses in understanding a situation as transitions occur (Benner *et al.*, 1999).

The importance of critical thinking for ophthalmic practice

One of the most important concepts emerging from these definitions is that of professional judgement. Nursing practice is driven by professional judgement, which is central to professional accountability and the provision of quality care. Critical thinking can help practitioners to enhance their skills of clinical judgement through developing better clinical understanding over time (Benner *et al.*, 1999).

Rolfe *et al.* (2001) suggest that developing the ability to think critically is now an essential component in the majority of educational programmes. Seymour *et al.* (2003) argue specifically that critical thinking is important for nursing for two reasons. Firstly, it relates to the growing body of nursing and related literature that practitioners have to make sense of and evaluate. Secondly, practitioners should be able to unmask or show the discrepancies between the values of their profession, the organisation in which they work, and what happens in practice. Seymour *et al.* (2003) further suggest that it is the applications of critical thought that are necessary to bring about change that is desirable for practice.

Applying critical thinking to ophthalmic practice

Applying critical thinking to ophthalmic practice is important. Benner *et al.* (1999) suggest that by being critical the practitioner is encouraged to move through a transition from a poorer to a better understanding. They provide the example of a cardiac surgical patient. In this situation, the fact that the practitioner can establish that the patient's low cardiac output is related to reduced circulating blood volume rather than cardiac pump failure can influence the ensuing nursing interventions and their expected outcomes.

Being critical is about asking questions related to practice. For example, a practitioner can ask questions about the changes taking place in a patient's condition. Such questions might be: Is the patient's level of consciousness lighter? Is there a trend towards an increased or decreased urine output? How do we account for the patient's weight gain? What are the patient's baseline observations?

THINKING POINT

TAKE A FEW MINUTES TO BECOME MORE AWARE OF THE WAY IN WHICH YOU THINK CRITICALLY.

A patient appears to be quite distressed and confused. She complains that her vision has suddenly become poor, and indicates she has developed a severe headache and is feeling very nauseated.

What questions would you ask about the signs and symptoms that this patient is presenting? Could this patient be having an acute glaucoma attack?

Now analyse your critical thinking processes.

- Why have you asked such questions?
- What subsequent nursing actions would you provide?

The answers that emerged for you from the questions you raised in the above thinking scenario will have provided the basis for your clinical judgement about managing the patient with acute glaucoma. These answers will also have been underpinned by a critical thinking approach. As Benner *et al.* (1999) argue, a good clinician should always be thinking critically about the present clinical situation and interpreting it in terms of the immediate past condition of the patient.

Reasoning-in-transition

'Reasoning-in-transition' refers to practical reasoning where a clinician takes account of the gains and losses in understanding a situation as transitions occur. Practical reasoning is also part of being critical in practice. But how does the process of reasoning-in-transition translate into practice? An example of this is a situation where the practitioner is caring for a post-operative patient recovering from a general anaesthetic. Here, the practitioner realised that the patient's high blood pressure was related to pain and not to vasoconstriction, or the effects of anaesthetic gases. Initially, however, the practitioner might have thought that the patient's hypertension was related to the anaesthesia, or because the patient was cold and vasoconstricted. Restoring the blood pressure back to normal by the administration of an intramuscular analgesic confirmed for the practitioner that the high blood pressure was pain-related.

THINKING POINT

THIS TIME, TAKE A FEW MINUTES TO TEST YOUR PRACTICAL REASONING AS AN OPHTHALMIC PRACTITIONER.

Imagine that you are preparing an ophthalmic patient to undergo an intravenous fluorescein angiography investigation. Prior to the procedure you realise that the patient is very irritable and is uncooperative.

Now consider the stages you would take to resolve this situation through your reasoning processes.

- What questions will you ask yourself?
- How will the answers to such questions enable you to make an accurate clinical judgement about the most appropriate course of action to take in order to regain the patient's cooperation?

In the above scenario, the ophthalmic practitioner would probably have reasoned that the patient's irritability and lack of cooperation were due to an impending hypoglycaemic attack, and not to the fear of having to undergo the procedure. To resolve this situation, the patient would have been given a glucose drink and something to eat. Initially, however, the ophthalmic practitioner might have thought that the patient's irritability was associated with increased anxiety levels, or extreme fears about having to have an intravenous injection in the arm. On regaining the patient's cooperation following the glucose drink and something to eat, the practitioner could confirm that her reasoning had been accurate in this situation by concluding that the irritability was due to hypoglycaemia.

Reflection, reflective practice and clinical narratives

A major challenge for ophthalmic practitioners will be to become an inquiring and insightful community to enable the achievement of improvements in healthcare delivery for the twenty-first century. Transforming practice can be achieved through insight and reason, but it will require a combination of the skills to reflect in practice,   alongside those of critical thinking when addressing practice issues (Price, 2004).

Reflection enables nurse practitioners to become meta-cognitive (White, 1999). This means practitioners gaining a better understanding of themselves in terms of their motives, perceptions, attitudes, values and feelings associated with the conduct of care (Taylor, 2003). This is important because practitioners work with the perceptions of other people and the meanings they ascribe to health, illness, signs and symptoms, and treatment. Self-awareness is the basis for being more open to understanding other people's perceptions. Reflection can help practitioners to view practice in a new light and challenge the assumptions they bring to it (Rolfe et al., 2001). Reflection can also encourage practitioners to discuss with others how any practice situation might be approached differently (Johns and Freshwater, 1998).

Clinical narrative reflection

Taylor (2003) argues that the premise of reflective practice is that nurses use a narrative about care, specifically of their own experiences, that enables them to appreciate episodes in a sensitive way. This translates into a process known as clinical narrative reflection. Through the writing of narratives about episodes in care, this process also becomes a means of developing critical thinking skills. Jasper's (1999) study confirmed that nurses identified the process of writing as facilitating critical thinking because it invited them to explore their experiences from different viewpoints (cited in Rolfe *et al.*, 2001). Clearly, experience is an important basis for critical thinking. Lomax and Parker (1996) argue that experience suggests that in order to explain what we know as practitioners, we have to describe the practice in which the knowledge is grounded in a 'living' form and content.

Developing the skills of narrative reflection is helpful in developing expert clinical judgement because reflecting on personal narrative reasoning can often reveal faulty logic such as tunnel vision or snap judgements (Benner *et al.*, 1999). Narratives can encourage an ophthalmic practitioner to give a first-person account of a critical incident that has occurred in practice. Such a narrative could include the practitioner's concerns, hunches, dialogue, changes in understanding over a period of time, and unresolved problems.

Benner *et al.* (1999) argue that a practitioner should tell the story to include the fears, risks, opportunities, and satisfactions experienced in order to uncover the practitioner's practical knowledge and the critical thinking processes used to achieve this. Narratives can offer ophthalmic practitioners the possibility of demonstrating clinical inquiry in practice. They help practitioners to identify clinical and ethical concerns, together with nursing knowledge, skills, and gaps in their knowledge that become evident from the story. Detailed narratives can contain clinical knowledge that has not yet been articulated in the ophthalmic nursing literature. Once the narrative has been written, the main themes can be analysed either individually or with other ophthalmic practitioners. In this way, it provides a forum for allowing ophthalmic practitioners to ask questions about their clinical practice and the ethical, clinical, and scientific reasoning behind it. Importantly, the implications of such an approach include developing sound clinical judgement and leadership skills, and advancing ophthalmic knowledge.

Research in ophthalmic practice

Research in ophthalmic practice

The development of critical thinking and reflective skills can also provide the platform for asking and formulating research questions. This is the basis for a fertile research culture. Undertaking more ophthalmic nursing research for the future is vitally important in striving to improve the delivery of high quality ophthalmic care. It also contributes to the evidence base, promotes innovation and accountability, and helps in risk management (Waterman, 2005). From a recent review of the literature, Waterman (2005) found that only 45 research papers worldwide had been published since 1997. However, ophthalmic practitioners can make a difference to patient outcomes and are at the forefront of the modernisation of the National Health Service in the UK.

Waterman (2005) has proposed a new strategy for improving the research culture by involving nurses, healthcare providers and health education institutes. The model consists of the following components:

- Take part in research when appropriate
- Make research part of career development and appraisal
- Link to researchers in their organisation
- Take part in studies and help establish priorities
- Link between healthcare providers and health education institutes to develop an R&D strategy
- Record nurses' skills, participation and output of research
- Provide resources and access to IT
- Make research part of a corporate plan
- Appoint a nursing research leader who can link with the health education institute
- Health education institutes (HEIs) must develop a programme of research and secure funding
- HEIs need to work with healthcare providers to provide R&D priorities, development and training.
- HEIs need to publish more research.
- HEIs need to work with healthcare providers to develop career pathways and provide research support.

The biggest challenge for ophthalmic practitioners is to convince others that they can undertake research and demonstrate effective skills in securing funding. Clearly, education is the key to success. The link between education and evidence-based practice is acknowledged and well documented in the educational and health and social care literature (Howarth and Kneafsey, 2005). Education, from undergraduate level onwards into continuing professional development, is needed to equip future practitioners with the skills to access, assess and use best evidence (Clough, 2002). Education will also enable competent, experienced ophthalmic and general nurse practitioners to contribute to nursing research. Such practitioners will be able to make astute and accurate observations and raise questions about their observations.

This view is also shared by Lancaster (2005) who argues that practitioners should consider the practice-based research models that enable bonding between education and practice through research. Lancaster (2005) suggests that the most reasonable model for bonding education and practice through research is collaborative research. This is regarded as research in which university-based researchers and agency-based clinicians collaborate as equal contributors at each stage of the research process. Team members draw on one another's expertise as they collaborate to achieve a successful clinical research study. Research is difficult to carry out in the absence of other colleagues. Collaborative practice-based research may be offered as a viable model for ophthalmic practitioners and researchers to engage in more ophthalmic research for the future. Ophthalmic practitioners need to collaborate on the research project with the appropriate university faculty from the onset. This involves mutually agreeing a research topic, developing the research method and data collection strategies, planning the data analysis method, writing the report and then disseminating the findings (Lancaster, 2005).

Research Governance Strategy

Importantly, when collaborating in research projects for the future, ophthalmic practitioners will need to meet the required standards of research practice. This is currently referred to as research governance. Governance is the system of administration and supervision through which research is managed, participants and staff are protected, and accountability is assured (Shaw *et al.*, 2005). For ophthalmic practitioners, this means being well informed about the government's Research Governance Strategy. This is known as the Research Governance Framework for Health and Social Care (DoH,2005). Its purpose is to promote excellence in research quality and mirrors clinical governance. It seeks to ensure that patients receive clinically effective, evidence-based care. It sets in place mechanisms for ensuring that research complies with all professional, ethical, legal, and scientific standards. This ensures good practice, and reduces adverse incidents (Shaw *et al.*, 2005). The framework reflects EU regulations and sets out the responsibilities of the individuals and organisations involved in research. This includes funders, researchers, organisations employing researchers, and healthcare organisations. Importantly, gaining approval for a research study is vital although problematic since different regulatory and approval bodies have different remits and agendas (Shaw *et al.*, 2005). Different bodies employ differing definitions of research to reflect their particular agendas and priorities. For example, distinctions are made between pure and applied research, biomedical and psychosocial, wet and dry research. Nevertheless, NHS research ethics committees are now required to deliver decisions following application within 60 days. Such committees are also being encouraged to move towards a culture of quality assurance and facilitation, as opposed to the policing of research (Shaw *et al.*, 2005).

Clinical governance

Undertaking future clinical research and caring for patients in a way that is evidence-based will continue as an important cornerstone of clinical governance (DoH, 1998, 2000). Equally, keeping up-to-date with government policies that will undoubtedly influence professional knowledge and clinical developments is also part of clinical governance and will be an ongoing challenge for ophthalmic practitioners.

Ophthalmic practitioners need to be cognisant of the sizeable body of literature that has emerged over the past eight years that embodies the government's vision for an effective and efficient patient-centred health service as part of a modernising agenda. The modernisation process was heralded by the government (DoH, 1997), and the constant challenge for ophthalmic practitioners is a high quality service provision (DoH, 1998, 2000). This strategy for reform has now been developed further in more recent government policies (DoH, 2001a, DoH, 2001b, DoH, 2003). Significantly, achieving the goals of the quality agenda will constitute the main targets for clinical ophthalmic practice. Already, in response to government policy health professionals' roles have been evolving and will continue to do so for the foreseeable future.

Conclusion

This chapter has discussed some important issues that influence the relationship between professional knowledge and evidence-based practice. These issues will continue to challenge the ophthalmic nursing community for the twenty-first century. Throughout this chapter continuing professional education was seen to be the key to success. It was seen to be instrumental in enabling ophthalmic practitioners to keep up-to-date with their professional knowledge and clinical developments, and develop critical thinking skills, supported by a commitment to reflective practice. Specifically, it was seen to foster research awareness, develop research knowledge, and provide the critical appraisal skills required to critique research evidence. This is important as a basis for making decisions about the suitability and feasibility of utilising research evidence in practice. Furthermore, continuing professional education can help to foster a spirit of inquiry and equip practitioners with the cognitive and practical skills to undertake clinical research in ophthalmic practice.

Within the overarching frameworks of clinical governance and research governance ophthalmic practitioners will be accountable for continually improving the quality of their clinical services and safeguarding high standards of care. The maintenance of professional accountability is grounded in sound clinical judgement about the need for evidence-based practice in order to achieve the highest standards of care. Moreover, clinical judgement can only become sound through ongoing development of professional knowledge and skills. This will provide ophthalmic practitioners with the confidence necessary to make effective decisions on their journey towards achieving excellence in ophthalmic care for the future. Thus, the main concepts addressed around professional knowledge and evidence-based ophthalmic practice will now be revisited in the final chapter's summary of the main issues impacting on the ophthalmic practitioner's future role in the delivery of a high-class ophthalmic service for the twenty-first century.

References

Benner, P. (1984). *From Novice to Expert*. California: Addison Wesley.

Benner, P., Hooper-Kyriadis, P., and Stannard, D. (1999). *Clinical Wisdom and Interventions in Critical Care. A Thinking-In-Action Approach*. Philadelphia: W.B. Saunders Company.

Brookfield, S.(1997). *Developing Critical Thinkers*. Milton Keynes: Open University.

Bryar, R., Closs, S., and Baum, G. (2003). 'The Yorkshire BARRIERS project: diagnostic analysis of barriers to research utilisation.' *International Journal of Nursing Studies* **40**: 73–85.

Clough, E. (2002). 'Putting governance into research and development.' *British Journal of Clinical Governance* **7** (1): 7–9.

Department of Health (1997). *The New NHS: Modern, Dependable*. London: The Stationery Office.

Department of Health (1998). *A First Class Service: Quality in the New NHS*. London: The Stationery Office.

Department of Health (2000). *The NHS Plan: A Plan for Investment, A Plan for Reform*. London: The Stationery Office.

Department of Health (2001a). *Investment and Reform in NHS Staff*. London: The Stationery Office.

Department of Health (2001b). *NHS Plan Implementation Programme*. London: The Stationery Office.

Department of Health (2003). *Improvement, Expansion and Reform: Priorities and Planning Guidance (2003-2006)*. London: The Stationery Office.

Department of Health (2005). *Research Governance Framework for Health and Social Care*. 2nd edn. London: Department of Health.

Dunn, V., Crichton, N., Roe, B., Seers, K., and Williams, K (1998). 'Using research for practice: a UK experience of the Barriers Scale.' *Journal of Advanced Nursing* **27**: 1203–10.

Ennis, R. (2001). *Outline of goals for a critical thinking curriculum and its assessment*. Available at: http://www.criticalthinking.net/goals.html (last accessed 23 February 2009).

Eraut, M. (1999). *Developing Professional Knowledge and Competence.* London: The Falmer Press.

Eraut, M. (2000). 'The intuitive practitioner: a critical overview.' In *The Intuitive Practitioner*, Atkinson, T., and Claxton, G. eds. Buckingham: Open University Press, pp. 255–68.

Facione, P. (2007). *2007 Update. Critical Thinking: What it is and why it counts.* CA: California Academic Press, pp. 1—23. Available at: http://www.insightassessment.com/pdf files/what&why98.pdf (last accessed 23 February 2009).

Gerrish, K., and Clayton, J. (2004). 'Promoting evidence-based practice: an organizational approach.' *Journal of Nursing Management* 12: 114–23.

Higgs, J., and Jones, M. (2000). 'Will evidence-based practice take the reasoning out of practice?' In *Clinical Reasoning in the Health Professions* 2nd edn, Higgs, J. and Jones, M. eds. Oxford: Butterworth Heineman, pp. 307–15.

Higgs, J., and Titchen, A. (2000). 'Knowledge and reasoning.' In *Clinical Reasoning in the Health Professions.* 2nd edn, Higgs, J. and Jones, M. eds. Oxford: Butterworth Heineman, pp. 23–32.

Howarth, M., and Kneafsey, R. (2005). 'The impact of research governance in healthcare and higher education organizations.' *Journal of Advanced Nursing* 49 (6): 675–83.

Hutchinson, A.M., and Johnston, L. (2004). 'Bridging the divide: a survey of nurses' opinions regarding barriers to, and facilitators of, research utilization in the practice setting.' *Journal of Clinical Nursing* 13 (3): 304–15.

Jasper, M. (1999). 'Assessing and improving student outcomes through reflective writing.' In Rust, C. (ed.) *Improving Student Learning – Improving Student Learning Outcomes.* Oxford: Oxford Centre for Staff Development, ch. 1.

Johns, C., and Freshwater, D. (1998). *Transforming Nursing through Reflective Practice.* Oxford: Blackwell Science.

Lacey, A. (1994). 'Research utilisation in nursing practice – a pilot study.' *Journal of Advanced Nursing* 19: 987–95.

Lacey, A. (1996). 'Facilitating research-based practice by educational intervention.' *Nurse Education Today* 16: 296–301.

Lancaster, J. (2005). 'Bonding of nursing practice and education through research.' *Nursing Educational Perspectives* 26 (5): 294–9.

Lomax, P., and Parker, Z. (1996). 'Representing a dialectical form of knowledge within a new epistemology for teaching and teacher education.' Paper presented at AERA, New York, April.

McLauchlan, R., Harker, R., MacDonald, H., Waterman, C., and Waterman, H. (2002). 'Using research to improve ophthalmic nursing care.' *Nursing Times* 98 (27): 39–40.

Parahoo, K. (2000). 'Barriers to, and facilitators of, research utilisation among nurses in Northern Ireland.' *Journal of Advanced Nursing* 31: 89–98.

Price, A. (2004). 'Encouraging reflection and critical thinking in practice.' *Nursing Standard* 18 (47): 46–52.

Rolfe, G., Freshwater, D., and Jasper, M. (2001). *Critical Reflection for the Nursing and the Helper Professions – a User's Guide.* Basingstoke: Palgrave Macmillan.

Sackett, D.L., Richardson, W.S., Rosenberg, W., and Haynes, R.B. (1997). *Evidence Based Medicine. How to Practice and Teach EBM*. Edinburgh: Churchill Livingstone.

Seymour, B., Kinn, S., and Sutherland, N. (2003). 'Valuing both critical and creative thinking in clinical practice: narrowing the research-practice gap?' *Journal of Advanced Nursing* 42 (3): 288–96.

Shaw, S., Boynton, P., andGreenhalgh, T. (2005). 'Research governance: where did it come from, what does it mean?' *Journal of the Royal Society of Medicine* 98 (11): 496–502.

Taylor, C. (2003). 'Narrating practice: reflective accounts and the textual construction of reality.' *Journal of Advanced Nursing* 42 (3): 244–51.

Upshur, R.E.G. (2001). 'The status of qualitative research as evidence.' In *The Nature of Qualitative Evidence*, Morse, J.M., Swanson, J.M., and Kuzel, A.J. (eds). Thousand Oaks CA: Sage, pp. 5–26.

Walsh, M. (1997). 'Perceptions of the barriers to implementing research.' *Nursing Standard* 11: 34–7.

Waterman, H. (2005). *Ophthalmic Nursing Research: Chronic Neglect Prompts Grim Diagnosis*. Paper presented at the Moorfields Hospital Bicentenary Scientific Meeting, February. London: Moorfields Eye Hospital.

Watkinson, S. (2001). *Exploring the relationship between nurses' perceptions of knowledge and research-based practice*. University of Surrey. PhD Thesis (unpublished).

White, C. (1999). 'The meta cognitive knowledge of distance learners.' *Open Learning* 14 (3): 37–46.

Chapter 11
Conclusion
Susan Watkinson

The future of ophthalmic practice
Professionalism
Evidence-based ophthalmic practice
Legal and ethical issues
Reflection, critical thinking skills and advanced practice
A plan for the future

Introduction

This final chapter will now reflect on the current issues and perceived future challenges presented in the preceding chapters of this book and attempt to integrate them into some strategies for the future. These strategies are presented initially as a conceptual diagram (see Figure 11.1). Each of the strategies portrayed in the diagram represents a response to the major challenges that will impact on the future of ophthalmic practice and that will need to be addressed.

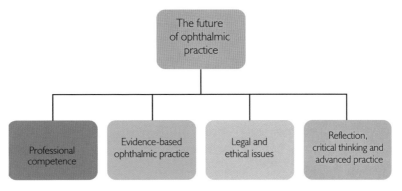

Figure 11.1   **The future of ophthalmic practice**

Professionalism

This chapter advances the view that ophthalmic practitioners need to adopt an overarching strategy that addresses how to become more decisive about developing their professionalism. An integral part of this is the maintenance of professional competence. Competence, however, is more than the acquisition of knowledge and skills to perform the task. It is also more than the acquisition of appropriate attitudes and the demonstration of professional behaviour. It also requires intrinsic motivation and a commitment to participation in continuing professional education.

Ophthalmic practitioners will need to develop a much larger professional body as a basis for widening their objectives and evidence-based strategies. Developing political awareness and demonstrating strong leadership will help to raise their professional profile. This in turn will help them to become more assertive and political in arguing the case for more resources for ophthalmic practice. A commitment to life-long learning will be instrumental in achieving this. The political clout to be gained through articulating their increasing knowledge of government healthcare policies, legal and ethical issues, professional developments, evidence-based practice, critical appraisal skills and the ability to critique and implement research evidence cannot be underestimated.

Evidence-based ophthalmic practice

The discourse of EBP dominates the current political agenda primarily as a justification for government spending on health care, but also as a means of identifying best clinical evidence. Technology appraisals remain the key source for accessing what is perceived as the best available evidence for the delivery of the most cost-effective and best clinical practice (NICE, 2008). Ophthalmic practitioners will clearly benefit from becoming evidence-based practitioners through an increased understanding of the different sources of evidence informing practice and through development of critical appraisal skills to assess the reliability and validity of research evidence. Such skills provide a basis for more informed decision-making about the need for utilising such evidence in practice.

An understanding of the role and use of advanced technology such as OCT (Optical Coherence Tomography) which permits non-invasive, high-quality, three-dimensional images of the retinal layers to aid management of age-related macular degeneration, and HRT (Heidelberg Retinal Tomography) to aid early glaucoma detection and management, is important. Such technology provides best evidence for decision-making about diagnosis and treatment, resulting in more effective client care. Knowledge of information technology and the development of information retrieval skills will also be instrumental in widening the knowledge base of research, increasing research awareness, and generally developing a research culture. This should also provide a springboard for participating in clinical research.

Legal and ethical issues

Legal and etical issues

Professionalism is also underpinned by the ability to deal with the growing complexities of daily ophthalmic clinical practice. This requires moral thinking and legal knowledge. Ophthalmic practitioners have a responsibility to ensure they are up-to-date with current law and professional ethical values. This forms a basis for exercising professional accountability within their specialist area of practice. Sound professional judgement is vital, but this does require that ophthalmic practitioners have knowledge of some legal concepts such as duty of care, informed consent, patients' rights, and more specifically for ophthalmic practice, organ donation and the Human Tissue Act 2004. The robust application of ethical and legal principles results in the delivery of better quality of care and is one of the hallmarks of advanced practice.

Reflection, critical thinking skills and advanced practice

Reflection

As highlighted in Chapter 10, ophthalmic practitioners need to become an inquiring community to enable improvements in healthcare delivery for the twenty-first century. Transforming practice is achievable through reason and insight, but it also requires a combination of skills to reflect in practice, coupled with those of critical thinking when addressing practice issues (Price, 2004). These are some of the hallmarks of advanced practice.

Being able to draw upon different kinds of knowledge enables the advanced nurse practitioner to develop critical and analytical skills. Critical thinking is self-regulatory judgement that results in demonstrating the ability to interpret, analyse, evaluate and infer. It demonstrates the ability to explore evidence, concepts, methods, and the criteria or contexts upon which that judgement is based (Facione, 2007). Reflection enables metacognition and this results in better self-awareness and self-understanding in relation to motives, perceptions, attitudes, values and feelings associated with the conduct of care (Taylor, 2003). Reflection can help ophthalmic practitioners to view practice in a new light and challenge the assumptions they bring to it (Rolfe *et al.*, 2001). In turn, this provides opportunities for making changes in their approaches to practice situations and advancing practice generally. The role of the advanced ophthalmic practitioner for the future will not be fulfilled unless knowledge, experience and research are translated into practice to change and improve it (Mantzoukas and Watkinson, 2007).

Thus, Mantzoukas and Watkinson (2007) summarise the generic features of advanced practice as being:

- the use of knowledge in practice
- critical thinking and analytical skills
- clinical judgement and decision-making skills
- professional leadership and clinical inquiry
- research skills
- changing practice.

An understanding of these generic features of advanced practice would facilitate ophthalmic practitioners, educators and clinical managers to develop those skills that would allow them to practice at an advanced level.

Before proceeding to a plan for the future, you are invited to reflect on the summary of key issues presented in this final chapter and consider their significance in the light of the Darzi report recommendations (DoH, 2008).

THINKING POINT

DO YOU FEEL READY TO SUPPORT AND CONTRIBUTE TO THE DARZI REPORT'S AGENDA?

Lord Darzi points out that tomorrow's clinicians are expected to commit to core principles, which will inform all planned changes for the planning and delivery of care (DoH, 2008, p. 8). These core principles include:

- focus on quality
- patient-centred care
- clinically driven
- flexibility
- valuing people
- life-long learning.

These core principles are all very relevant and will undoubtedly continue to impact on the ophthalmic nursing community for the twenty-first century. Clearly, Lord Darzi paints a compelling and inspiring portrait of the modern nurse as one rooted in the values of the nursing profession and the NHS. Caring is re-defined as trying to meet the modern requirements of personalisation and choice. Care is delivered by practitioners who plan and provide care, are advocates and guardians of the quality of care and promoters of good health for people and communities (DoH, 2008, p. 18).

A plan for the future

A plan for the future

The ophthalmic community of practice lives in interesting times. The climate is one of excitement as well as frustration. However, the ophthalmic community needs to embrace any future challenges. It needs to take what is best from the present, which are the core values of caring for patients, together with what is best from the emerging future, which is a knowledge-driven, rapidly advancing technological society. There then needs to be a marrying of the present with the future to create something far greater than both for the practice of ophthalmic nursing. In trying to decide how to face the current and future challenges discussed throughout this book perhaps the ophthalmic practitioner should hold a glass of water in front of her and ask herself: Is this glass half empty or half full? The answer to this question will surely be significant in determining the future direction of ophthalmic practice.

> ## THINKING POINT
>
> TAKE A FINAL PAUSE FOR THOUGHT
>
> As a practitioner, are you now ready to face the current issues and address the future challenges of ophthalmic practice?

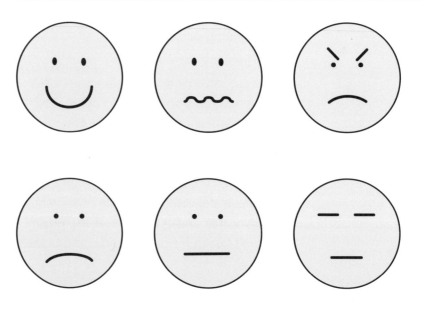

Figure 11.2

Which of the above emotions are you now identifying with?

Conclusion

In the final analysis, the outcome of addressing these strategies for the future will be an enhanced ability to demonstrate the application of an advancing knowledge base to practice and an increased level of competence and confidence on the journey towards achieving clinical excellence in ophthalmic practice.

References

Department of Health (2008). *High Quality Care for All: NHS Next Stage Review Final Report*. London: DoH.

Facione, P. (2007). *2007 Update. Critical Thinking: What It Is and Why It Counts.* CA: California Academic Press. pp.1–23.
Available at: http://www.insightassessment.com/pdf_files/what&why98.pdf
(last accessed 23 February 2009)

Mantzoukas, S., and Watkinson, S. (2007). 'Advanced nursing practice: reviewing the international literature and developing the generic features.' *Journal of Clinical Nursing* 16 (1): 28–37.

National Institute of Clinical Excellence (2008). *Technology Appraisals.* www.nice.org.uk (last accessed 22 November 2008).

Price, A. (2004). 'Encouraging reflection and critical thinking in practice.' *Nursing Standard* 18 (47): 46–52.

Rolfe, G., Freshwater, D., and Jasper, M. (2001). *Critical Reflection for the Nursing and Helper Professions – a User's Guide*. Basingstoke: Palgrave Macmillan.

Taylor, C. (2003). 'Narrating practice: reflective accounts and the textual construction of reality.' *Journal of Advanced Nursing* 42 (3): 244–51.

Index